CHILDREN AND *Violence*

CHILDREN AND

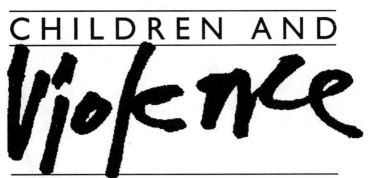

Violence

EDITED BY DAVID REISS, JOHN E. RICHTERS,
MARIAN RADKE-YARROW, & DAVID SCHARFF

THE GUILFORD PRESS

NEW YORK / LONDON

Published by The Guilford Press
A Division of Guilford Publications
72 Spring Street, New York, NY 10012

© 1993 The Washington School of Psychiatry
Published simultaneously as
Psychiatry: Interpersonal and Biological Processes,
Volume 56, Number 1, February 1993.

ISBN 0-89862-588-2

Last digit is print number: 9 8 7 6 5 4 3 2 1

Printed in the United States of America

Contributors

CARL C. BELL, MD, Department of Psychiatry, University of Illinois School of Medicine; Community Mental Health Council, Inc., Chicago.

MARILYN BENOIT, MD, Department of Psychiatry, Children's National Medical Center; Department of Psychiatry and Behavioral Sciences and Pediatrics, George Washington University, Washington, DC.

DANTE CICCHETTI, PhD, Mt. Hope Family Center, Department of Psychology, University of Rochester, New York.

ROBERT N. EMDE, MD, University of Colorado Health Sciences Center, Denver.

ANA C. FICK, PhD, Louisiana State University Medical Center, New Orleans.

BERNARD Z. FRIEDLANDER, PhD, Department of Psychology, University of Hartford, West Hartford, Connecticut.

NORMAN GARMEZY, PhD, Professor Emeritus, Department of Psychology, University of Minnesota, Minneapolis.

ESTHER J. JENKINS, PhD, Department of Psychology, Chicago State University; Community Mental Health Council, Inc., Chicago.

DELLA M. HANN, PhD, Louisiana State University Medical Center, New Orleans.

RAYMOND P. LORION, PhD, Department of Psychology, University of Maryland, College Park.

MICHAEL LYNCH, Mt. Hope Family Center, Department of Psychology, University of Rochester, New York.

PEDRO MARTINEZ, MD, Laboratory of Developmental Psychology, National Institute of Mental Health, Bethesda, Maryland.

JOY D. OSOFSKY, PhD, Louisiana State University Medical Center, New Orleans.

FRANK W. PUTNAM, MD, Laboratory of Developmental Psychology, National Institute of Mental Health, Bethesda, Maryland.

MARIAN RADKE-YARROW, PhD, Laboratory of Developmental Psychology, National Institute of Mental Health, National Institute of Health, Bethesda, Maryland.

DAVID REISS, MD, Department of Psychiatry and Behavioral Sciences, George Washington University, Washington, DC.

JOHN E. RICHTERS, PhD, Child and Adolescent Disorders Research Branch, National Institute of Mental Health, Rockville, Maryland.

WILLIAM SALTZMAN, MA, University of Maryland, College Park.

DAVID SCHARFF, MD, Washington School of Psychiatry, Washington, DC.

PENELOPE K. TRICKETT, PhD, Department of Psychology, University of Southern California, Los Angeles.

SARAH WEWERS, MEd, MSW, School Board Saint Charles Parish Public Schools, Luling, Louisiana.

Contents

Introduction: American Violence and Its Children

David Reiss

This special issue is devoted to a major crisis in American social life: the rapid rise of serious physical violence in the public and private spaces of our communities. The 12 papers in this issue document the rise in violence and grapple with comprehending its impact on children's physical, psychological, and social development. Three themes, all emphasizing urgency, are expressed by these papers.

First, crude statistics – such as arrest records and murder rates – are serving as a loud alarm about the increase in the incidence of violent acts in many American communities. However, a clear picture of the implications of this violence for children requires much *better information on the kinds of violent acts to which children are exposed*. We need to know whether they are the physical victims of violence, whether they have observed it or just heard about it. We need to know the patterns and duration of their exposure, and to learn about factors that increase some children's exposure, within a community, and factors that protect other children. In short, we need to supplement police statistics with epidemiological investigation that is sensitive to both community dynamics and developmental processes. The papers by Richters and Martinez and that by Osofsky and her colleagues are the first to delineate and carry through investigations of this kind. The paper by Bell and Jenkins summarizes some of the work of their influential Chicago group in this area.

A second theme is the special necessity to take what we know now and begin to build *strategies for intervention*. The paper by Lorion and Saltzman spells out an imperative to take some remedial action to protect children before epidemiologic and developmental investigation has provided a blueprint of the problem that is clear by conventional scientific standards. As these authors emphasize, research projects that are conducted in volatile, stigmatized, and dangerous communities are themselves interventions: they place a special burden on the investigator to both study and be a responsible part of the community and its processes. The paper by Bell and Jenkins also takes us beyond simple observation of violence and its effects to monitoring the impact of an innovative intervention program. A similar process is exemplified by the Friedlander paper. Here, the encouragement of violent behavior by violent television is placed in the context of a broader set of concepts about the causes of violence. This placement, in turn, illustrates that television is just one of many influences promoting violence; it may even have a paradoxical effect of keeping a child at home and away from danger outside. Indeed, this paradoxical effect of television seems to open the way for another: that the power of television may be even greater to influence constructive and protective behavior. The Friedlander paper sketches some of the dimensions of a program to use media as a protective intervention against violence and for supporting socially constructive behavior.

David Reiss, MD, is Editor of *Psychiatry*; he is with George Washington University.

Third, the urgent need for information now – to improve research and to bring us quickly to effective intervention – requires us to *search in closely related fields for ideas and data*. Putnam and Trickett provide a summary of important data on the impact of child sexual abuse on psychological development in childhood and adolescence, and even some of its long-term effects in adult life. While Putnam and Trickett clarify that there are some differences between community violence, particularly in public places, and sexual abuse, they provide a fascinating summary of evidence focusing on two important processes that may mediate the impact of abuse on development: the psychological process of dissociation and biological processes in the adrenal and gonadal hormone systems. In a similar vein, Cicchetti and Lynch draw on their extensive studies of child maltreatment – often in the family setting – as well as data from other centers. They show how these data can contribute to understanding the impact of community violence on children. In a carefully elaborated model they delineate risk and protective factors in cultural, community, family, and individual developmental processes, and show how they influence the emergence of competence and psychopathology in children.

Taken together, these nine papers clarify the need for integrating information now available. The reader who carefully reviews their important observations will appreciate the integrative papers at the close of this issue. Emde's paper heightens our awareness of a central developmental crisis: How do children develop a core or implicit sense of morality in a culture of violence? Benoit ponders the impact of violence from the perspective of an experienced clinician. Garmezy closes the issues with a reasoned exploration of factors accounting for the resilience of children faced with severe adversity and provides an impassioned plea for the deployment of this country's resource to support the potential for resilience in the children and families who currently face the worst.

The papers in this issue were first presented at the National Conference on Community Violence and Children's Development: Research and Clinical Implications. The conference was jointly sponsored by the National Institute of Mental Health, the John D. and Catherine T. MacArthur Foundation, Research Network Award, and *Psychiatry* along with its parent organization, the Washington School of Psychiatry. The conference was initiated by the Laboratory of Developmental Psychology in the Intramural Research Program under the guidance of Marian Radke-Yarrow and John Richters, and by the Editorial Board of this journal under the guidance of Robert Emde, associate editor. Detailed planning was carried out by Radke-Yarrow, Richerts, and David Scharff, director of the Washington School. These papers thus, reflect, in part, a journalistic activism appropriate for an urgent problem. We encourage a comparable activism in our readers. Please write to give us your response to these papers and to convey your ideas about additional work that is important in this field. If there are a sufficient number of letters we will publish them in a special section along with responses from authors of these papers.

Community Violence and Children's Development: Toward a Research Agenda for the 1990s

John E. Richters

THE UNITED STATES is the most violent country in the industrialized world—particularly for young people. Homicide in the United States ranks as the second leading cause of death among those between 15 and 24 years of age (Earls et al. 1991). Males, especially, are at high risk. As indicated in Figure 1, those between 15 and 24 years of age were more likely to be murdered than their counterparts in all 22 other developed countries for which comparable homicide statistics were available during 1986–1987 (Fingerhut and Kleinman 1990). Young males were 4 times more likely to be murdered than their counterparts in the next highest country, Scotland; 7 times more likely than young males in Canada; 21 times more likely than those in West Germany; and 40 times more likely than same-age males in Japan. Moreover, the U.S. homicide rate for Black males (15 and 24 years) was more than 7 times the homicide rate for White males in this age range. These figures are all the more alarming in light of the fact that homicide rates in major U.S. cities have increased steadily since these data were recorded.

Firearms account for the majority of homicides among teens and young adults (Centers for Disease Control 1988; Christoffel and Christoffel 1986; Jason 1983). Since the mid-1980s firearms have accounted for 96% of the increase in U.S. homicide rates (Centers for Disease Control 1990) and have become a staple of childhood and teenage life in many American cities. In a few short years the widespread availability and use of handguns has transformed childhood into something quite foreign to what most adults can recall of their own childhoods. In urban school districts around the country, school dress codes have given way to metal detectors, hall monitors have given way to armed security patrols, and school yard spats over minor injustices have given way to murders and drive-by shootings.

In the midst of this transformation the public health community has focused its attention on the years of potential life lost due to violence (Centers for Disease Control 1988), the associated economic costs to the nation (Wintemute and Wright 1990), and efforts to reduce the number of injuries and deaths associated with the growing violence (Public Health Service 1990). Relatively little attention, however, has been focused on the causes of this surge in violence, or on the psychological consequences to individuals and families of living in what are often chronically and desperately violent circumstances.

John E. Richters, PhD, is with the Child and Adolescent Disorders Research Branch of the National Institute of Mental Health.

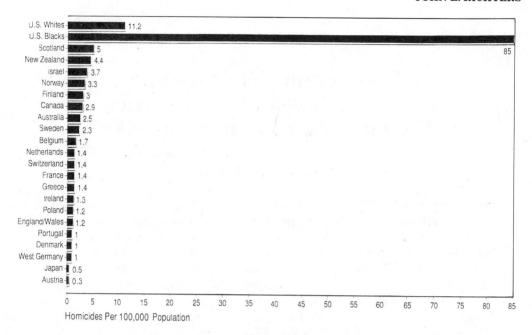

Figure 1.
International variation in homicide rates for males 15 through 24 years of age in 1986 or 1987. Data sources: National Center for Health Statistics, World Health Organization, and country reports. Modified from Fingerhut and Kleinman (1990).

It is clear from the contributions to this special issue of *Psychiatry* that the fields of psychiatry and psychology have much to contribute to the study of community violence and children's development. But it is also clear that the scientific community is at a considerable disadvantage in trying to estimate the full scope of the community violence problem and its implications for children and families. The professionals most familiar with the phenomenon and with the populations most affected tend not to have the training, skills, or motivation to study the problem systematically. As a consequence, we are left with little beyond police statistics and newspaper reports of violence levels as crude indices of the magnitude of the problem. Thus, there is a clear and urgent need for intensive, community-based epidemiological research designed initially to identify the children most at risk for exposure to violence in the community as either victims or witnesses, and to assess the consequences of that exposure in terms of so-cial-emotional adjustment problems and psychopathology. Equally important are questions concerning individual, family, and community factors that function to protect children from exposure, and, once exposed, to shield them from the untoward consequences of that exposure.

A number of specific research priorities are implicit within this general framework. For example, very little is known about which types of violent experiences pose the greatest threat to adaptive social and emotional functioning in children. Clearly, not all violent experiences hold the same threat value (Cicchetti 1991). Therefore, delineating which types of violent experiences in different contexts pose the greatest threat deserves a high priority in studies of community violence. A taxonomy of violence exposure will also be indispensable to developing and implementing intervention strategies by identifying populations and individuals at greatest risk for maladjustment and psychopathology following exposure.

The fields of psychology and psychiatry are in a much better position to operationalize the domains of social-emotional and psychiatric adjustment that deserve emphasis in study of community violence effects on children. Research and theory on posttraumatic stress disorder (Pynoos et al. 1987), children living in war-torn areas of the world (Jensen and Shaw in press), and children raised in violent families (Cicchetti and Toth 1992) point to numerous domains of cognitive, social, emotional, and psychophysiological functioning that can be severely affected by exposure to violence, including depression, withdrawal, extreme fear, anxiety, affect disregulation, blunted affect, dissociative reactions, aggression, intrusive thoughts, and flashbacks. And standardized measures have been developed for assessing many of these domains, ranging from clinically important individual differences within the normal range to diagnosable psychopathology.

But despite these gains, there is much that we still do not know. For example, which types of symptoms/reactions to violence exposure are normative and/ or transient, with few if any implications for subsequent development, and which symptoms/reactions have implications for long-term development? The media have focused repeatedly in recent years on the apparent indifference of some young children to wounded and dead bodies at crime scenes in the wake of violence. To what extent does this reflect a normal, adaptive response to repeated violence exposure? To what extent and under what circumstances might this putative indifference be pathological in the sense that it is likely to generalize to a broader indifference to human suffering? What are the psychological and biological processes implicated? To what extent does such apparent indifference signal a child's diminished recognition of danger, perhaps placing the child at greater risk for engaging in risk-taking behavior that otherwise would be avoided? What types of interventions might be developed and tested to prevent such a process from unfolding? And beyond relatively immediate reactions, how might children's exposure to violence in the community influence their ability to experience and modulate states of emotional arousal, their images of themselves, their beliefs in a just and benevolent world, their beliefs about the likelihood of surviving into adulthood, their willingness to form affective relationships with those who may not survive the violence, the value they place on human life, their sense of morality, and a range of other topics central to normal/adaptive development. These issues define the boundaries of a broad and important research agenda for studying the consequences of community violence for children's development. It is our hope that the papers in this special issue of *Psychiatry* will kindle sufficient interest, concern, and activity in the scientific community to advance our understanding of these issues.

REFERENCES

CENTERS FOR DISEASE CONTROL. Biometrics Branch, Division of Injury Epidemiology and Control, Center for Environmental Health and Injury Control. Premature mortality due to homicides: U.S., 1968–1985. *Morbidity and Mortality Weekly Report* (1988) 37:543–45.

CENTERS FOR DISEASE CONTROL. Homicide among young black males–United States, 1978–1987. *Morbidity and Mortality Weekly Report* (1990) 39: 869–73.

CHRISTOFFEL, K. K., and CHRISTOFFEL, T. Handguns as a pediatric problem. *Pediatric Emergency Care* (1986) 2:75–81.

CICCHETTI, D., ed. Defining psychological maltreatment. Special issue: *Development and Psychopathology* (1991) 3:1–124.

CICCHETTI, D., and TOTH, S., eds. *Child Maltreatment Child Development, and Social Policy.* Norwood, NJ: Ablex, 1992.

EARLS et al. Position paper: Panel on prevention of violence and violent injuries. Solicited by the Division of Injury Control, Centers for Disease Control. Paper presented at the third annual National Injury Control Conference, Atlanta, GA, April 1991.

FINGERHUT, L. A., and KLEINMAN, J. C. International and interstate comparisons of homicide among young males. *Journal of the American Medical Association* (1990) 263:3292–95.

JASON, J. Child homicide spectrum. *American Journal of Delinquency and Crime* (1983) 137: 573–81.

JENSEN, P. J., and SHAW, J. Children as victims of war: Current knowledge and future research needs. *Journal of the American Academy of Child and Adolescent Psychiatry*, in press.

PYNOOS, R. S., FREDERICK, C., NADER, K., AR- ROYO, W., STEINBERG, A., ETH, S., NUNEZ, F., and FAIRBANKS, L. Life threat and posttraumatic stress in school-age children. *Archives of General Psychiatry* (1987) 44:1057–63.

PUBLIC HEALTH SERVICE. *Healthy People 2000: National Health Promotion and Disease Prevention Objectives.* U.S. Department of Health and Human Services, 1990.

WINTEMUTE, G. J., and WRIGHT, M. Initial and subsequent hospital costs of firearm injuries. *Archives of Surgery* (1990).

The NIMH Community Violence Project: I. Children as Victims of and Witnesses to Violence

John E. Richters and Pedro Martinez

THE 1980s WITNESSED an extraordinary increase in community violence in most major cities across the United States. In 1990 the homicide rate in Boston increased by 45% over the previous year; in Denver, by 29%; in Chicago, Dallas, and New Orleans, by more than 20%; in Los Angeles, by 16%; in New York, by 11%. In Washington, DC, which has the highest per capita homicide rate in the country, the 1990 murder rate set an all time record in the District's history (Escobar 1991). Across the country, 1 out of 5 teenage and young adult deaths was gun related in 1988 – the first year in which firearm death rates for both Black and White teenagers exceeded the total for all natural causes of death combined. Also in 1988, the firearm homicide rate for young Black males increased by 35%, and Black male teens were 11 times more likely than their White counterparts to be killed by guns (Christofel 1990).

Although the murder rate itself has received nationwide attention and concern, it represents only a crude index of the day-to-day community violence that characterizes many neighborhoods throughout American cities. Increasingly, children have been involved both as victims of and eyewitnesses to episodes of community violence. In Washington, DC, for example, even school-based violence has become so common that many school principals in the District have banned students from wearing coats or carrying bookbags during class hours, for fear that they may be carrying weapons (Sanchez and Horwitz 1989). Between September of 1988 and January of 1989, 20 area students were wounded by gunshots or knives on or near their school grounds. In December 1988 two students were wounded by gunfire from a passing car as they left a DC high school; in January 1989 four students were wounded when two gunmen sprayed bullets into a crowd of several hundred

John E. Richters, PhD, is with the Child and Adolescent Disorders Research Branch of the National Institute of Mental Health.

Pedro Martinez, MD, is with the Laboratory of Developmental Psychology of the National Institute of Mental Health.

This research was supported by the National Institute of Mental Health and by a grant from the Early Childhood Transitions Network of the John D. and Catherine T. MacArthur Foundation. We thank Robert Emde, Marian Radke-Yarrow, and Peter Jensen for their encouragement and support throughout each phase of this research. We also thank Dante Cicchetti, Frank Putnam, and Marilyn Benoit for their contributions to the early development of this project. Finally, we thank the principal, teachers, staff, and families of the Southeast Washington, DC, elementary school (anonymous on request) in which this study was conducted.

Send requests for reprints to John Richters, Child and Adolescent Disorders Research Branch, Division of Clinical Research, National Institute of Mental Health, 5600 Fishers Lane, Room 10-104, Rockville, MD 20857.

students leaving another District high school, an incident sparked by a lunchtime argument in the cafeteria (Sanchez and Horwitz 1989); in March 1989 four children were wounded when two youths approached and sprayed shots at them without saying a word (Sanchez 1989). These are not isolated incidents. During the first eight months of 1988 an estimated 220 children and teenagers were wounded or killed by shootings in Washington, DC (Sanchez 1989). Shootings have become so commonplace that schools throughout Washington, DC, and in major cities across the country, have found it necessary to install metal detectors to prevent students from bringing weapons to class.

Despite the alarming portrait of community violence depicted by police statistics and media coverage, there has been little systematic research into the nature and consequences of children's exposure to violence in urban communities. The need for such a research agenda is clear. It is only by identifying children most at risk for exposure and its consequences – including psychopathology, physical injury, and death – that public health agencies and services delivery systems can target their scarce resources. And it is only on the basis of such risk/exposure information that preventive intervention programs aimed at reducing exposure and its consequences can be effectively designed, implemented, and evaluated. Beyond these immediate needs lie a host of equally pressing theoretical questions concerning the consequences of being raised in violent environments in the shaping of various dimensions of personality development and the emergence of psychopathology.

The study described here was an initial effort to (1) assess the extent to which young children living in a moderately violent inner-city community had been exposed both directly (as victims) and indirectly (as witnesses) to various forms of violence, and (2) examine the extent to which these exposure patterns are related to characteristics of the children and their families.

METHOD

Subjects

The primary sample included 165 children, ages 6 to 10 years, living in a low-income, moderately violent neighborhood in Southeast Washington, DC. All children attended the same elementary school (K–6); 111 children attended first and second grades, the remaining 54 children attended the fifth and sixth grades. Information concerning children's violence exposure was elicited independently from the children and their parents (typically their parents). In addition, teachers rated the stability and violence levels of homes of all children in their classes, including those who did not participate in the study. Thus, teacher-informant data were collected on all children attending grades 1 and 2 ($n = 152$), and 5 and 6 ($n = 88$); parent-informant and/or child-informant data were collected from 111 (73%) of the first- and second-grade, and 54 (61%) of the fifth- and sixth-grade children.

Procedures

Recruitment letters describing the study were sent home to the parent(s) of all children attending grades 1, 2, 5, and 6. The letters were printed on school letterhead and were cosigned by the school principal and investigators. The study was described as an effort to document the extent to which the children had been exposed, directly and indirectly, to different forms of violence in the community. Teachers then contacted parents directly to answer questions about the study, encourage participation, and schedule appointments for visits to the school for interviews. Upon their arrival at school, parents were greeted by the investigators, who explained the study in detail and secured informed consent. In light of the literature on experimenter/interviewer effects on respondents, particularly those associated with race (Sattler 1970), parents were told explicitly not to either exaggerate or conceal instances of violence to which their children had been exposed; they were told that the success of the study depended on total honesty from respondents. Then, depending on their reading skills, parents either completed the assessment battery with minimal assistance from, or responded to an oral administration of the assessment battery by, one of the investigators. All parents were paid $20.00 cash for their participation.

Children were then surveyed by the investigators in small groups during school hours in a reserved classroom. Teachers completed their measures following parent and child participation. Children and teachers also were told explicitly not to either exaggerate or conceal instances of violence to which the children had been exposed, and that the success of the study depended on total honesty.

Parent-Completed Measures

All parents completed the parent report version of the Survey of Children's Exposure to Community Violence (Richters and Saltzman 1990), which assesses the frequency with which an index child has been victimized by, has witnessed, or has heard about 20 forms of violence and violence-related activities in the community (explicitly *not* including media exposure; see Table 3). For each positive response, the questionnaire includes context questions about (1) where the violence took place (in or near school versus home), (2) who perpetrated the violence (ranging from stranger to family member), (3) who, if not the child, was victimized (ranging from stranger to family member), and (4) when the incident occurred (ranging from 1 week ago to more than 5 years ago). Parents also completed the Conflict Tactics Scales (Straus 1979), a widely used questionnaire for assessing within-family violence between adults. In addition, parents completed a questionnaire concerning a variety of characteristics of family history, composition, and demographics.

Child-Completed Measures
(Grades 1 and 2)

Children completed *Things I Have Seen And Heard* (Richters and Martinez 1990a), a 15-question structured interview that probes young children's exposure to violence and violence-related themes in an age-appropriate format. The interview consists of 15 pages, each describing a different form of violence/violence themes. As shown in Figure 1, five stacks of balls are depicted below each description of violence, each with a different number of balls, ranging from none to four; the columns are labeled sequentially from "never" to "many times." Prior to administration, children were taught how to circle the stacks to indicate frequency of exposure. As each violence description was read aloud, children were asked to circle a stack of balls indicating how often they had either witnessed or had been victimized by that form/theme of violence. The 1-week test–retest reliability of the composite variable reflecting the sum of all instances of child reported exposure was $r = .81$ for a random subsample of 21 children, with a small, nonsignificant attenuation in the absolute levels of exposure reported at time 2, $t(20) = 1.34$, ns.

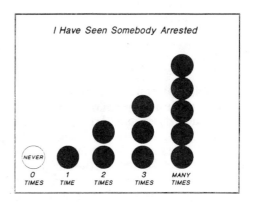

Figure 1.
Sample drawing of violence exposure questions from "Things I Have Seen and Heard" asked of younger children (grades 1 and 2).

Child-Completed Measures
(Grades 5 and 6)

Fifth- and sixth-grade children were assembled in small groups to complete the self-report version of the Survey of Children's Exposure to Community Violence (Richters and Saltzman 1990). Again, depending on their reading and comprehension skills, children either completed the assessment battery with minimal assistance or responded to an oral administration of the assessment battery by an investigator.

Teacher-Completed Measure

Teachers completed the Teacher Observation of Classroom Adaptation (TOCA-R — Werthamer-Larsson, Kellam, Dolan, Brown, and Wheeler 1990). The TOCA-R includes 43 classroom problems of children, including internalizing and externalizing behaviors. Each behavior is rated on a six-point Likert scale, reflecting the frequency with which it is manifest by the child. In addition, teachers were asked to what extent each child's home was characterized by stability and violence. Both additional questions also were rated on six-point Likert scales. Analyses of the teacher TOCA ratings of classroom adaptation are not included in this report.

RESULTS

Sample Characteristics

As indicated in Table 1, the families of the younger and older children did not differ significantly on any of the major demographic characteristics assessed. The majority of participating parents had not completed high school. Fifty-four percent of the parents in both the younger and older sample were employed full time; the median family income was less than $19,000, with one quarter of the families receiving some form of public assistance. The majority of parents were not cur-

rently married, and almost 50% had never been married. As a consequence, more than 50% of the children had rarely or never lived with their biological fathers.

Comparison of participating and nonparticipating families. The availability of teacher ratings of nonparticipating as well as participating children and families provides a basis for estimating the extent to which participation in the study was systematically associated with characteristics of either the children or their families. The results of these comparisons are presented in Table 2.

As indicated, there were no significant differences in teacher-rated family violence and family stability between participating and nonparticipating families for either age group. Moreover, children of participating and nonparticipating families did not differ significantly on teacher ratings of classroom-based behavior problems or overall student progress. There was, however, a nonsignificant trend toward higher levels of teacher-rated behavior problems among children of nonparticipating families in the younger sample. This trend did not, however, hold for children in the older sample.

Neighborhood violence level. Data concerning the prevalence, frequency, and correlates of children's exposure to violence are most interpretable in the context of figures concerning actual levels of neighborhood violence. Such data allow for comparisons across studies and support the computation of violence/exposure-risk estimates for prevention, intervention, and policy planning initiatives. Figure 2 reflects the levels of reported violent crimes for each of the seven wards[1] in Washington, DC, during 1989, the year immediately preceding the study.[2]

As indicated, the study school was located in a moderately violent ward (Ward 7) in comparison with other areas of the

---

[1]The wards represent multicensus track geographical areas of the District with approximately equal population densities.
[2]Data supplied by the District of Columbia Criminal Justice Plans and Analysis Unit, 1990.

Table 1

SAMPLE CHARACTERISTICS

Respondent Characteristics	*Samples*	
	Grades 1/2 (%)	Grades 5/6 (%)
Relationship to child:		
Biological mother	79	80 ns
Biological father	9	10 ns
Other relative	12	10 ns
High school graduate/GED	36	26 ns
Employed full time	54	54 ns
Marital status		
Currently married	17	16 ns
Never married	46	43 ns
Race: African American	97	96 ns
Family		
Income <$19,000	57	49 ns
Receiving some public assistance	26	27 ns
Living in apartment	67	64 ns
Child		
Males	51	52 ns
Females	49	48 ns

Note. All demographic differences between families of younger and older children were nonsignificant.

District; violence in Ward 7 was just below the median level of reported violence across all seven District wards. Thus, the results reported here are not a consequence of sampling in an unusually violent community within the District, although community violence levels in Ward 7 were nonetheless high by conventional (i.e., middle-class, suburban) standards.

Table 2

COMPARISON OF PARTICIPATING AND NON-PARTICIPATING FAMILIES BASED ON TEACHER RATINGS OF FAMILIES AND CHILDREN

Teacher-Rated Characteristic *Younger Children*	*Family Participation Status*			
	Participating (*n* = 78)	Non-Participating (*n* = 35)		
	Mean (SD)	Mean (SD)	t *value*	p
Family stability	3.13 (1.75)	2.66 (1.63)	1.35	.18
Family violence	2.40 (1.60)	2.17 (1.27)	0.74	.46
Child behavior problems	102 (25.97)	110 (25.00)	1.70	.09
Student progress	2.78 (1.46)	2.69 (1.43)	0.33	.74
Older Children	(*n* = 52)	(*n* = 35)		
	Mean (SD)	Mean (SD)	t *value*	p
Family stability	4.22 (1.47)	4.10 (1.78)	0.32	.75
Family violence	3.24 (1.83)	3.24 (2.04)	0.01	.99
Child behavior problems	128 (33.65)	127 (35.36)	0.03	.97
Student progress	2.76 (1.15)	3.03 (1.56)	0.93	.36

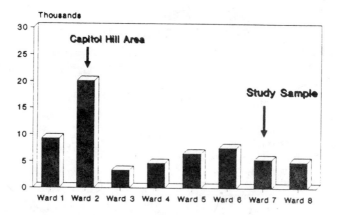

Figure 2.
Reported violence in Washington, DC, 1989: comparison of study
ward (7) with other wards in the District. Data supplied by the
Washington, DC, Criminal Justice Plans and Analysis Unit.

Patterns of Community Violence Exposure

Parents' reports. The prevalence rates for children being victimized by and witnessing each form of community violence according to parents' reports are presented in Table 3; prevalence rates are reported separately for younger and older children.

For initial comparison purposes, all categories of violence exposure were collapsed into two categories: direct victimization by violence and witnessing violence to others. The resulting variables reflect the proportion of children who had been victimized by or had witnessed at least one instance of violence in the community. Across all forms of violence, parents' reports indicated that children were significantly more likely to report having witnessed violence to someone else than to have been victimized themselves. These significantly higher rates of witnessing than victimization held for children in both the younger (84% vs. 21%, $p < .001$) and older (90% vs. 35%, $p < .001$) groups. As indicated in Table 3, however, there are more ways to witness violence to others than to be victimized oneself (e.g., witnessing a dead body, witnessing a killing, witnessing someone carrying an illegal

weapon). The data presented here therefore examine differences between the prevalence rates for victimization and witnessing across a standard set of violence categories; namely, those for which it was logically possible to be victimized directly and to witness violence to someone else, including shootings, stabbings, muggings, sexual assaults, threats of serious physical harm, being approached about illegal drug use, being approached about drug dealing, forced entries. The following data therefore *underestimate* the actual prevalence rates for witnessing violence.

Victimization vs. witnessing. Both younger and older children were significantly more likely to have witnessed violence directed at someone else than to be victimized themselves. Whereas 19% of the younger children had been victimized by some form of violence in the restricted set of categories, 61% had witnessed violence to someone else ($\chi^2(1) = 30.41$, $p < .001$. This difference was accounted for by higher rates of witnessing stabbings (13% vs. 1%, $p < .01$), muggings (25 vs. 9%, $p = .01$), threats of physical harm (17% vs. 5%, $p = .02$), and illegal drug use (53% vs. 1%, $p < .001$). Similarly, whereas 32% of the older children had been victimized by some form of violence, 72% had witnessed violence to someone else, $p < .001$. This

Table 3

PARENTS' REPORTS OF THEIR CHILDREN'S COMMUNITY VIOLENCE EXPOSURE

	Prevalence Rates			
	Grades 1 and 2		Grades 5 and 6	
Violence Category	(n = 77)		(n = 51)	
	Victim (%)	Witness (%)	Victim (%)	Witness (%)
Shooting	3	9	6	14
Stabbing	1	13	4	4
Sexual assault	0	1	2	4
Mugging	9	25	8	43
Physical threat	5	17	14	18
Approached: drug trade	4	5	6	12
Approached: drug use	1	53	4	61
Arrest[a]	—	37	—	20
Punch/hit/slap[a]	—	39	—	38
Illegal weapon[a]	—	18	20	
Forced entry: other	3	5	6	10
Forced entry: own[a]	—	5	—	0
Dead body outside[a]	—	16	—	16
Murder[a]	—	3	—	4
Suicide[a]	—	0	—	3

[a]Victimization question not asked and/or not logically possible.

difference was accounted for among older children by a significantly higher rate of witnessing muggings (43% vs. 8%, $p <$ .001) and illegal drug use (61% vs. 4%, $p < .001$).

Between-age differences. Across the restricted set of violence categories, older children were somewhat, though not significantly, more likely than younger children to be victimized by (32% vs. 19%, $\chi^2(1) = 2.34$, ns) and to witness (72% vs. 61%, $\chi^2(1) = 1.27$, ns) community violence. Nonetheless, individual comparisons reveal that older children were significantly more likely than younger children to have witnessed both muggings (43% vs. 25%, $\chi^2(1) = 4.80, p < .05$) and arrests (70% vs. 37%, $\chi^2(1) = 14.37, p < .001$).

Across all forms of violence, there was a nonsignificant tendency for parents to report a higher prevalence of victimization by violence among older compared to younger children (35% vs. 21%, $\chi^2(1) = 3.31, p = .07$. Thus, although older children suffered rates of victimization in particular violence categories that were some-

times double the rate for younger children, the absolute rates in each group were sufficiently low to fall well short of statistical significance.

Within-family violence. The parents' responses on the Conflict Tactics Scales (CTS – Straus 1979) indicate that a significant number of the children's homes were characterized by relatively high levels of violence between adults. The proportions of families in which adults used each form of physical violence in the home during the previous year are shown in Figure 3. As indicated, the prevalence rates for both minor and severe violence in the study sample were between 5 and 6 times the national average based on population survey data collected in 1985 (Straus and Gelles 1990).

Younger children were not probed about violence exposure within the family. Older children, however, were asked a single question about how often they had been victimized by and had witnessed slapping, hitting, and punching within the family. We compared these responses with a summary variable reflecting the highest level of family violence reported by parents. Across all families, the older children's reports of victimization and witnessing violence in the family were not significantly related to maternal reports of family violence level. This lack of association is influenced strongly by two factors. First, a subset of parents ($n = 5$) reported that they *never* engaged in any of the conflict resolution strategies described in the CTS, including discussing issues calmly; their failure to endorse any resolution tactics may, therefore, reflect an unwillingness to disclose any information about conflict resolution within the family. Second, 51% of the children reported never having experienced or witnessed slapping, hitting, or punching within the family. For the subset of families in which the children reported any violence and the parents endorsed any method of conflict resolution, their agreement on the relative level of family violence was strong and significant, $r(14) = .67, p < .01$.

Teachers responded to two single-item questions concerning the violence level and stability of the children's homes. Across all families of younger children, teachers' reports of family violence and stability were not significantly related to parents' reports. For the subset of families in which parents endorsed any form of conflict resolution, however, agreement between teachers and parents was low but significant, $r(60) = .32, p = .01$.

Older Children's Reports

The prevalence rates for victimization and witnessing community violence based on the older children's reports are presented in Table 4 according to type of violence. Consistent with parents' reports, significantly more older children reported having witnessed violence to others than having been victimized themselves (97% vs. 59%), $\chi^2(1) = 14.45, p < .01$. Moreover, among the subset of families for whom both parent and child reports were available, significantly more older children reported having been victimized by

some form of violence than was indicated by their parents' reports (69% vs. 44%), $\chi^2(1) = 4.59, p < .05$. Follow-up analyses, however, revealed that boys reported significantly higher rates of victimization than girls (88% vs. 25%), $\chi^2(1) = 14.44, p < .01$, accounting entirely for the higher rates of victimization reported by children compared to parents. In contrast, the prevalence of witnessing community violence based on the older children's reports was identical to the rate reported by their parents (75%). These prevalence estimates, however, are based on group-level comparisons of parents' and children's reports. Pairwise agreement between parents and their children is examined below.

Parent–child agreement about exposure. Composite violence exposure variables were created separately for parents' and children's reports by summing across all reports of victimization by and all reports of witnessing community violence. Pairwise comparisons of parents' and children's reports based on these summary variables revealed sex-related differences in parent–child agreement about violence exposure. Moderate agreement held between boys and their parents for both victimization, $r(18) = .39, p = 11$, and witnessing, $r(18) = .51, p < .03$ violence, although agreement reached significance only for witnessing violence due to the small sample size. In contrast, agreement between girls and their parents was poor for both victimization, $r(17) = .16$, ns, and witnessing violence, $r = .98$, ns. Inspection of the bivariate scatterplots revealed that these sex differences in parent–child agreement are not attributable to sex-related range differences. Finally, children and parents were about equally likely to report having heard the sound of gunfire in their neighborhoods (74% vs. 61%). Pairwise agreement between parents and children about how often they had heard gunfire in their neighborhoods was moderately high and significant, $r(35) = .51, p < .01$. Again, agreement was substantially lower for girls ($r = .27$) than boys ($r = .47$), but neither of these separate estimates reached significance due to sample size ($n = 24$).

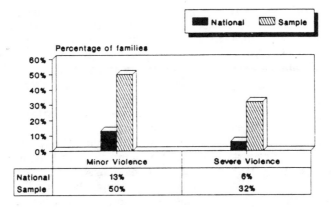

Figure 3.
Prevalence rates of within-family violence reported by parents,
comparison of sample and national norms. Based on 1985 population resurvey (Straus and Gelles 1990).

Location of violence exposure. For each instance of violence exposure, older children were asked whether the event took place in the home, near home, in school, or near school. According to children's reports, none of the victimization events took place in their homes, although 48% of the reported victimization took place somewhere *near* their homes. In contrast, 22% of the victimization, according to

children's reports, took place in school, and the remaining 30% took place *near* school. Thus, the older children were slightly more likely to be victimized by violence in or near school (55%) than near their homes (48%), although the difference was small and nonsignificant.

The majority of violence witnessed by the older children took place near their homes (68%), with 22% of the incidents

Table 4

OLDER CHILDREN'S REPORTS OF COMMUNITY
VIOLENCE EXPOSURE

($n = 37$)

Community Violence Categories	Victim (%)	Witness (%)
Shootings	11	31
Stabbings	0	17
Muggings	22	43
Sexual assaults	6	3
Physical threats	47	22
Drug trade	9	67
Drug use	0	22
Arrests	11	74
Punch/hit[a]	—	44
Weapon[a]	—	58
Chased by gang	37	39
Forced entry	3	14
Dead bodies[a]	—	23
Woundings[a]	—	29
Murders[a]	—	9
Suicides[a]	—	3

[a]Victimization question not asked and/or not logically possible.

15

taking place in school. A relatively small proportion of the violence witnessed by the older children took place in their homes (7%) or in school (9%).

Involvement of family and friends. Older children were asked also whether each instance of victimization and witnessing violence involved family members, friends, acquaintances, and/or strangers. According to the children's reports, a relatively small proportion of victimization events were perpetrated by family members (13%). But the majority were committed by those familiar to the children (friends 50%; acquaintances 12%), whereas only 25% of the events were perpetrated by strangers. Similarly, the majority of violence witnessed by the children was committed by those familiar to them (family 21%, friends 25%, acquaintances 16%); in contrast, 38% of the violence witnessed was committed by strangers. Victims of violence witnessed by older children were similarly distributed. The majority of victims were known to the children (family 13%, friends 38%, acquaintances 16%), whereas 38% of the victims were strangers.

Frequency of exposure. Table 5 presents the distributions of exposure frequency for each category of violence according to the older children's reports. Consistent with the prevalence rates for exposure, witnessing violence to others was generally more common than direct victimization. For example, 22% of the older children reported witnessing illegal drug use almost every day, whereas being approached about drug use was a relatively uncommon event, occurring as often as once a month for only 3% of the children. Similarly, 15% of the children reported having witnessed a mugging or beating 7 or 8 times, whereas none reported having themselves been victimized by a mugging or beating more than 3 or 4 times. These data are most useful in underscoring the fact that the prevalence rates reported earlier do not, for most categories of violence, reflect exposure to single, isolated events. Finally, composite variables reflecting the total frequency of both victimization by and witnessing violence were significantly associated for boys, $r(18) = .52$, $p < .05$, but not for girls, $r(17) = .11$, ns.

Younger Children's Reports

The reports of first- and second-grade children about their violence exposure are more difficult than the reports of older children to compare with their parents' reports; younger children were probed about exposure to only a limited set of violence categories, using an age-appropriate response format that differed substantially from the one used by their parents. Among the categories probed, six were directly comparable with parents' reports,

Table 5

PREVALENCE RATES FOR YOUNGER CHILDREN'S
COMMUNITY VIOLENCE EXPOSURE: COMPARISON
OF PARENT AND CHILD REPORTS ABOUT
WITNESSING VIOLENCE

Prevalence Rates (%)

Violence Categories	Parent's reports	Children's reports	χ^2	p
Shootings	9	47	25.30	<.001
Stabbings	13	31	3.88	.05
Muggings	8	45	23.54	<.001
Arrests	57	88	17.40	<.001
Drug deals	53	69	3.54	.06
Dead body	16	37	7.63	<.001
Serious accidents	11	74	58.48	<.001

Table 6

FREQUENCY OF VICTIMIZATION BY AND WITNESSING[a] DIFFERENT FORMS OF COMMUNITY VIOLENCE

Number of Times

Categories of Exposure	Never	1	2	3 or 4	5 or 6	7 or 8	At Least Once a Month	At Least Once a Week	Almost Every Day
Shootings	89/70	8/8	/5	/8	3/3	/5			
Stabbings	100/84	/8	/5	/3					
Muggings	78/58	11/19	5/6	5/3			/6	/3	/3
Sexual assaults	95/97	/3				5			
Physical threats	54/78	16/8	5/3	11/8		8			5
Drug use	92/35	5/8	/14	/5		/8	3/	/8	/22
Drug Trade	100	/3	/3	/5		/3	/3		/5
Arrests[b]	−/28	−/17	−/8	−/8	/14	−/3	/3	/6	/14
Punch/hit[b]	−/57		−/16	−/8	/3	/3	/5		/3
Weapon[b]	−/43	−/19	−/14	−/11	/3	/5			/5
Chased by gang	64/62	6/19	6/11	14/5		/3	3/	6/	3/
Forced entry	97/91	/9	3/						
Dead bodies[b]	−/75		/14		/6	/3		/3	
Woundings[b]	−/72	−/11	−/17						
Murders[b]		−/91	−/3	−/3	−/3				
Suicides[b]	/97	/3							

[a]All numbers represent proportions of children responding positive to each frequency. Numbers before the slash represent the proportion for victimization; numbers following the slash represent proportions for witnessing.
[b]Victimization not asked and/or not logically possible.

including the witnessing of arrests, drug deals, muggings, shootings, stabbings, and encountering dead bodies outside.

As indicated in Table 6, younger children were significantly more likely than their parents to report that they had witnessed six out of seven types of violence. For more than half of these categories (shootings, muggings, stabbings, serious accidents) the children were between 2 and 6 times more likely than their parents to report having been witnesses to violence. These child-reported prevalence rates — particularly for witnessing muggings (45%), shootings (47%), stabbings (31%), and dead bodies (37%) — seem unusually high for 6- and 7-year-old children. Most of these rates, however, do not differ significantly from the rates reported by their older fifth- and sixth-grade schoolmates (muggings: 40%; shootings: 31%, dead bodies: 26%). The exception to this pattern is the number of younger children who reported having witnessed a stabbing (37% vs. 17% for the older children), $\chi^2(1) = 7.63, p < .01$.

Despite the sizable absolute discrepancies between parents' and younger children's reports of community violence exposure, their pairwise agreement concerning *relative* levels of exposure parallels the agreement patterns between older children and their parents. Separate summary variables were created for parents' and children's ratings of both victimization and witnessing by summing across all categories of violence. Agreement between boys and their parents based on these summary indices was moderate for both victimization, $r(26) = .38, p = .05$, and witnessing community violence, $r(26) = .42, p < .05$. In contrast, agreement between girls and their parents was poor for both victimization, $r(23) = .09$, ns, and witnessing, $r(23) = -24$, ns.

Mediators of Community Violence Exposure

Several demographic family characteristics were examined as possible mediators of risk for violence exposure, includ ing respondent's education, income level, marital status, and living arrangements. Both younger and older children's reports of total violence exposure were significantly associated only with family living arrangements. For example, younger children who reported higher levels of victimization by violence in the community were more likely to live in houses rather than apartments, $r(62) = .29$, $p < .05$, and to have lived for a longer period of time in their current dwellings, $r(62) = .25$, $p = .05$. Similarly, younger children who reported higher levels of witnessing violence in the community were more likely to live in houses rather than apartments, $r(62) = .34$, $p < .01$. Those who lived in houses also had moved less often during the past 5 years, $r(62) = -.26$, $p < .05$, and tended to have lived longer at their current addresses, $r(62) = .43$, $p < .01$.

The exposure context information provided by older children allowed for separate examinations of risk factors associated with violence involving those familiar to them versus those involving strangers. Results indicate a trend toward higher levels of exposure involving familiar persons among the children of less-educated parents, $r(33) = .33$, $p = .06$; this trend did not hold for exposure to violence involving strangers, $r(33) = .03$, ns. Conversely, exposure to violence involving strangers was significantly higher among children living in houses compared to apartments, $r(36) = .39$, $p < .05$; this association did not hold for exposure to violence involving those familiar to the children, $r(36) = -.03$, ns.

DISCUSSION

The data presented indicate clearly that, according to independent reports from children and their parents, both older and younger children in this sample had been exposed to relatively high levels of violence in their homes and neighborhoods. Although a disturbing number of younger and older children had been direct victims of violence, they were between 2 and 4 times as likely to witness violence to others and/or violence-related scenes involving others. Thus, although public health statistics concerning children (and adults) typically focus on direct victimization by violence (Christofel 1990), it is clear that *witnessing* violence by children also deserves attention as a public health issue. Although the psychological consequences of exposure are not yet known, there can be little question that merely being in the presence of violence places children in harm's way.

Although we found impressive test–retest reliability for reports of violence exposure among a random subsample of the younger children, the study did not afford an opportunity to examine text–retest reliability of reports from either parents or older children. However, our confidence in the ability and willingness of children and parents to provide useful estimates of violence exposure is buttressed by their group-level agreement, their moderate and significant levels of pairwise agreement, and by the details of violence exposure they often volunteered during face-to-face interviews. Moreover, the significant associations between summary exposure ratings based on parents' and their younger children's reports indicate that children as young as age 6 can provide useful information about violence exposure.

Nonetheless, the poor pairwise agreement between parents and their daughters in both the younger and older samples raises questions about who provided the most accurate reports. Among older children, we are inclined to place more credence in the children's reports for two related reasons. First, the children were asked to report about violence that they themselves had experienced. Parents, on the other hand, were dependent for their knowledge of most types of children's violence exposure on what their children had reported to them. It is therefore not surprising that discrepancies between their reports of violence exposure were almost always in the direction of children reporting more than did their parents. To an unknown extent this may have been due to children simply not reporting violence exposure to their parents. In some cases reporting to parents may result in restrictions in children's activities and/or unwanted monitoring and supervision. In other cases, the violence exposure may not be sufficiently salient to the children to warrant reporting to parents. Relatively common events such as drug deals in the neighborhood may lose their signal value and therefore not be reported to others.

Parent–child discrepancies in reporting may to an unknown extent also be due to parents repressing information about their children's violence exposure as an active or passive coping strategy. We have seen anecdotal evidence of this process in follow-up interviews with selected families and in videotaped interactions between the parents and their children, wherein some parents actively discouraged their children from talking about violence they had witnessed. But, regardless of its origin, the fact that parents so consistently underestimated their children's violence exposure is significant for several reasons. Obviously, lack of parental awareness may place parents at a disadvantage in their efforts to monitor and effectively supervise their children's activities. This disadvantage may decrease their effectiveness in protecting their children from subsequent violence exposure. Furthermore, the possibility that children may not be reporting more common forms of violence to their parents suggests that it may be beginning to lose its emotional impact for them. If true, this may have a range of important implications, not the least of which is the risk that desensitization may translate into a diminished ability to recognize and therefore avoid objectively dangerous situations and activities.

It is commonly believed that the likelihood of community violence exposure increases significantly when children begin attending school. Parents' reports of their children's violence exposure in this sample tend to confirm this expectation; their rat-ings indicate a trend toward higher levels of exposure for older compared to younger children. The reports of younger children themselves, however, suggest that a significant number of them had already witnessed high levels of violence by the time they entered first grade – significantly more so than indicated by their parents' reports. Moreover, those children with higher levels of violence exposure also reported significantly higher levels of distress symptoms.

Nonetheless, the absolute levels of exposure reported by the younger children were sufficiently high to raise questions about the veracity of their reports. Unfortunately, there is no absolute criterion against which to gauge the integrity of their reports. It is possible, of course, that the anonymity of responding in small groups may have engendered exaggerated response sets that would have been less likely in individual interviews. Moreover, younger children may have failed to discriminate sufficiently between violence that they had actually witnessed and violence that they had only heard about. We deliberately avoided requiring children to offer details of their exposure so as not to bias them against reporting violence they were uncomfortable talking about. In future research, it would be useful to probe for details of reported violence after all instances of exposure have been reported; such a procedure would allow researchers to explore the veracity of reports without risking such bias. In any event, whether one relies more on the reports of parents or their children, the present data suggest that efforts to study the cumulative effects of violence exposure on children will need to begin at very early ages.

As indicated earlier, we deliberately selected the study school because it is located in a moderately violent neighborhood according to DC police data on reported violent crimes. Nonetheless, we have no basis for estimating the extent to which patterns of exposure reported here are representative of other schools in the District of Columbia, let alone in other cities around the country. It is worth noting, however, that a comparison of reported violent crimes in this neighborhood with reported violent crimes in other major U.S. cities during the year preceding the study indicate that violence in the study neighborhood was near the median for other major cities.

We are somewhat more confident about the representativeness of participating families in this study to the population of families with children attending the same grades in the study school. According to teacher reports of family stability and violence, as well as their ratings of children's adjustment, there were no significant differences between the observed characteristics of participating compared to nonparticipating families and children. But this is a very limited set of potentially biasing characteristics and warrants expansion and scrutiny in future research.

Although the primary focus of the present study was on children's exposure to community violence, parents reported disturbingly high levels of violence between adults within their homes. Prevalence rates of both minor and severe violence were between 5 and 6 times the national average. These data underscore the importance of supplementing measures of community violence exposure with assessments of within-family violence. They also underscore the fact that some children in violent neighborhoods are raised in a subculture of violence beginning at home. Children raised in violent homes within violent neighborhoods are at an extraordinary disadvantage for normal development, underscoring the need to study the long-term consequences of chronic violence exposure on children's personality development. The high prevalence rates for within-family violence in this sample also have important implications for intervention programs designed to protect children from violence exposure and its consequences, because many such programs rely on working with parents who are not themselves the perpetrators of violence.

It warrants underscoring that the violence exposure survey instruments developed for this study yield only crude assays of the stimulus-rich violence to which the children had been exposed. They are a useful and necessary starting point for assessing violence exposure. But significant gains in our understanding of the consequences of exposure will require assessment strategies and instruments with a much higher degree of fidelity to violence phenomena and contexts than survey instruments afford. There are many types of shootings; they can result in wounds of many different types, body locations, and levels of severity; they can be witnessed at close proximity or at a distance; they can take place in contexts otherwise thought of as safe or dangerous; they can involve persons of different relationships to and with a child. All forms of violence can vary along these and other important dimensions. Thus, there is probably little basis for the simplifying assumption that witnessing a shooting will be more severe in its effects on a child than witnessing someone being chased or threatened. It therefore seems clear that research on the effects of acute and/or chronic violence exposure will require the development of a taxonomy of exposure that takes into account all these dimensions.

Finally, it should be noted that the limitations of sample size and the breadth/depth of our assessments precluded more than a cursory exploration of child and family factors associated with higher and lower levels of exposure to violence. To be sure, some of these differences in exposure are probably attributable to differences in the actual violence levels that characterize the children's neighborhoods. But it seems equally clear from our exposure interviews that children living on the same neighborhood blocks were often exposed to impressively different levels of violence. Thus, one of the most important goals for future research in this area should be the identification of personal as well as family and community factors associated with higher and lower levels of children's violence exposure.

REFERENCES

CHRISTOFEL, K. K. Violent death and injury in US children and adolescents. *American Journal of Disease Control* (1990) 144:697–706.

ESCOBAR, G. Washington area's 703 homicides in 1990 set a record. *Washington Post* (January 21, 1991), p. 1.

RICHTERS, J. E., and SALTZMAN, W. *Survey of Children's Exposure to Community Violence: Parent Report.* National Institute of Mental Health, 1990.

RICHTERS, J. E., and MARTINEZ, P. *Checklist of Child Distress Symptoms: Parent Report.* National Institute of Mental Health, 1990a.

RICHTERS, J. E., and MARTINEZ, P. *Things I Have Seen and Heard: A Structured Interview for Assessing Young Children's Violence Exposure.* National Institute of Mental Health, 1990b.

SANCHEZ, C. Four youngsters wounded in NE schoolyard shooting. *Washington Post* (March 21, 1989), p. 1.

SANCHEZ, R., and HOROWITZ, S. 4 wounded in gunfire at Wilson High. *Washington Post*, (January 27, 1989), p. 1.

SATTLER, J. M. Racial "experimenter effects" in experimentation, testing, interviewing, and psychotherapy. *Psychological Bulletin* (1979) 73:137–60.

STRAUS, M. A. Measuring intrafamily conflict and violence: The Conflict Tactics (CT) Scales. *Journal of Marriage and the Family* (1979) 41: 75–88.

STRAUS, M. A., and GELLES, R. J. *Physical Violence in American Families: Risk Factors and Adaptations to Violence in 8,145 Families.* Transaction Publishers, 1990.

WERTHAMER-LARSSON, L., KELLAM, S. K., DOLAN, L., BROWN, C. H., and WHEELER, L. *The Epidemiology of Maladaptive Behavior in First Grade Children.* Johns Hopkins University School of Public Health, 1990.

The NIMH Community Violence Project: II. Children's Distress Symptoms Associated with Violence Exposure

Pedro Martinez and John E. Richters

THE rising tide of violence in American cities has placed the causes and consequences of violence squarely on the public health agenda. The U.S. Government's *Year 2000 National Health Promotion and Disease Prevention Objectives* includes a full chapter devoted to violence issues and delineates a number of goals and programs aimed at reducing the number of deaths and injuries associated with violence (Public Health Service 1990). Notably absent from these objectives, however, is attention to the possible adverse psychological consequences of exposure to acute or chronic violence. Nonetheless, in light of numerous media reports of children's exposure to community violence and recent reports documenting high levels of exposure even among very young children (Richters and Martinez 1993), it is reasonable to question whether the risks of exposure extend beyond death and physical injury to psychological well-being.

Unfortunately, there has been no systematic research to date concerning the psychological consequences to children of being raised in chronically violent neighborhoods. Mainstream studies of stress and children's adjustment have focused on a variety of childhood stressors both within and outside the family. Prominent among within-family stressors have been factors such as bereavement (Brown, Harris, and Bifulco 1986), divorce (Emery 1982), parent psychopathology (Watt, Anthony, Wynne, and Rolf 1984), child abuse (Cicchetti and Rizley 1981; Frederick 1986), life stress (Compas 1987), and the like. There also have been less frequent reports over the decades concerning children's symptoms in the wake of natural disasters such as floods (Burke, Borus, and Burns 1986; Gleser, Green, and Winget 1981), tornadoes (Silber, Perry, and Bloch 1958), earthquakes (Galante and Foa,

Pedro Martinez, MD, is with the Laboratory of Developmental Psychology of the National Institute of Mental Health.

John E. Richters, PhD, is with the Child and Adolescent Disorders Research Branch of the National Institute of Mental Health.

This research was supported by the National Institute of Mental Health and by a grant from the Early Childhood Transitions Network of the John D. and Catherine T. MacArthur Foundation. We thank Marian Radke-Yarrow, Robert Emde, and Peter Jensen for their encouragement and support throughout each phase of this research. We also thank Frank Putnam and Dante Cicchetti for their contributions to the early development of this project, and Jean-Pierre Valla, who graciously permitted us to modify and build on his in-progress, cartoon-based psychiatric interview for use with young children (*Dominique*). Finally, we thank the principal, teachers, staff, and families of the Southeast Washington, DC, elementary school (anonymous on request) in which this study was conducted and Marilyn Benoit for facilitating this partnership.

Send requests for reprints to John Richters, Child and Adolescent Disorders Research Branch, Division of Clinical Research, National Institute of Mental Health, 5600 Fishers Lane, Room 10-104, Rockville, MD 20857.

1986), landslides (Lacy 1972), nuclear power plant accidents (Handford et al. 1986), and transportation accidents (Tuckman 1973), as well as their symptoms following kidnappings (Terr 1979, 1981, 1983), concentration camp experiences (Kinzie, Sack, Angell, Manson, and Rath 1986; Sack, Angell, Kinzie, and Rath 1986), familicide (Lebovici 1974), and a range of other violent and traumatic experiences (Garmezy and Rutter 1985). But perhaps most germane to the issue of community violence are the clinical literatures concerning effects on children of exposure to the chronically violent circumstances of war (McWhirter 1982, 1983; Rosenblatt 1983).[1]

CHILDREN'S REACTIONS TO WARTIME STRESS

Clinical-descriptive reports of children's reactions to wartime stress date back to World War II (Bodman 1941; Freud and Burlingham, 1943; Glover 1942), with more systematic studies appearing in the wake of the Yom Kippur War in Israel (Breznitz 1983; Milgram 1982; Milgram and Milgram 1976; Ziv and Israel, 1973); and during the ongoing conflict in Northern Ireland (Lyons 1973, 1979; McAuley and Troy 1983; McWhirter, 1982, 1983; McWhirter and Trew 1981). Reports of children's symptom patterns have varied considerably across studies as a function of the domains of adjustment targeted, stressors involved, age and sex of children, and other background characteristics of the samples studied. Generally, however, children's reactions associated with exposure to war-related violence have included intrusive thoughts, fear of

recurrence, anxieties, difficulty concentrating, depression, psychosomatic disturbances, sleep disturbances, and other symptoms that, in the extreme, have come to be associated with posttraumatic stress.

As Garmezy and Rutter (1985) observed in their excellent review of these and related studies, point estimates of psychiatric risk among children exposed to wartime stressors are difficult to judge due to the clinical-descriptive nature of many reports and inattention to methodological detail. Important information concerning baseline or prestressor symptom levels of children, the full range of stressors involved, and mediating conditions is often not reported, rendering comparisons across studies a difficult task. Consequently, there is little basis for reconciling the highly variable estimates of significant psychiatric symptoms in children; prevalence estimates have ranged from 10% to 50%. Nonetheless, it is clear that some children exposed to wartime stress do suffer socially handicapping emotional problems. Typically, however, it is impossible to determine from empirical reports whether their symptoms are reactions to particular stressors such as bombings (Ziv and Israel 1973), evacuations (John 1941), death/absence of a parent (Kinzie et al. 1986); or to the more generalized chronic violence and unpredictability of wartime conditions; or, more generally, to characteristics of the children's environments that are unrelated to war violence. Hence, the cumulative literature on children in wartime highlights an important problem but yields few systematic conclusions about children's immediate and long-term consequences to children of living in chronically violent circumstances, or about factors that mediate those reactions.

CHILDREN'S REACTIONS TO ACUTE VIOLENCE IN THE COMMUNITY

In perhaps the most systematic study of the effects of children's exposure to

---

[1]There is, of course, an enormous research literature concerning the effects on children of exposure to media violence. In contrast to living in chronically violent circumstances, however, viewing violence on television is a vicarious source of stimulation that children characteristically seek out, enjoy, and can easily escape. This literature therefore may have limited relevance to the present focus despite its potential as a source of influence on children.

community violence, Pynoos and his colleagues (Pynoos et al. 1987) recently reported on children's (grades K through 6) distress symptoms 1 month following a fatal schoolyard sniper incident in Los Angeles. Their report supports several conclusions. First, a host of children's distress symptoms covaried significantly with their levels of actual proximity to the shooting incident. Second, children who knew the deceased child reported more severe symptoms. Third, children who had experienced other traumatic events during the previous year reported having renewed thoughts and images of those events; many of their distress symptoms were related to both events. Finally, these effects held equally well for children as young as 6 years old.

The Pynoos et al. study provides compelling evidence for children's posttraumatic symptoms following exposure to an acute episode of urban violence. But the authors set out specifically to examine children's symptoms in response to a single, particularly traumatic violent incident. Their report does not, therefore, address important questions concerning (1) the long-term sequelae of exposure to *chronic* violence; (2) family, neighborhood, and children's own characteristics that may mediate their reactions—immediate and long-term, adaptive and maladaptive—to violence; or (3) the impact of violence exposure on characteristics of children's social and emotional functioning beyond those associated with distress.

Notwithstanding the limitations of earlier reports concerning children and violence, two common themes have emerged that are worthy of note. First, children who are exposed to violent incidents are significantly more likely than those not exposed to suffer from a wide range of social and emotional problems. Prevalence rates are not always as high as one might expect *a priori*, but they are certainly high enough to warrant concern about violence as a risk factor for children's adjustment. Second, characteristics of children's families and family relationships seem to be major mediators of both their short- and long-term adaptation in the wake of violence. This theme emerges strongly from reports concerning British children following bombing-related evacuations in Britain in World War II (Freud and Burlingham 1943) and more recently concerning traumatized Cambodian children who were relocated to the United States following their concentration camp experiences (Kinzie et al. 1986; Sack et al. 1986). It is not yet clear, however, whether similar exposure-distress reactions are characteristic also of children living in chronically violent urban neighborhoods. Nor is it clear to what extent distress reactions are associated more broadly with emotional and behavioral problems in children.

The data reported in this paper were drawn from the NIMH Community Violence Pilot Project. In our initial report, we described children's patterns of exposure to violence in their communities and families (Richters and Martinez 1993). In this report, we focus on reports from the children and their parents concerning symptoms of distress and fear associated with children's violence exposure.

METHOD

Subjects

The primary sample included 165 children, ages 6 to 10 years, living in a low-income, moderately violent neighborhood in Southeast Washington, DC. All children attended the same elementary school; 111 children attended the first and second grades, the remaining 54 children attended the fifth and sixth grades. Information concerning the children's violence exposure and distress symptoms was elicited independently from children and their parents.

As described in detail elsewhere (Richters and Martinez 1993), the majority of participating parents had not completed high school. Fifty-four percent of the parents in both samples were employed full time; the median family income was less than $19,000, with one quarter of the families receiving some form of public assistance. The majority of parents were not currently married, and almost 50% had never been married. As a consequence, more than 50% of the children had rarely or never lived with their biological fathers.

Procedures

Recruitment letters describing the study were sent home to the parent(s) of all children attending grades 1, 2, 5, and 6. The letters were printed on school letterhead and were cosigned by the school principal and investigators. The study was described as an effort to document the extent to which the children had been exposed, directly and indirectly, to different forms of violence in the community. Teachers then contacted parents directly to answer questions about the study, encourage their participation, and schedule appointments for visits to the school for interviews. Upon their arrival at school, parents were greeted by the investigators, who explained the study in detail and secured informed consent. In light of the literature on experimenter/interviewer effects on respondents, particularly those associated with race (Sattler 1970), parents were told explicitly not to either exaggerate or conceal instances of violence to which their children had been exposed; they were told that the success of the study depended on total honesty from respondents. Then, depending on their reading skills, parents either completed the assessment battery with minimal assistance from or responded to an oral administration of the assessment battery by an investigator. All parents were paid $20.00 cash for their participation.

Children were then surveyed by the investigators in small groups during school hours in a reserved classroom. Children also were told explicitly not to either exaggerate or conceal instances of violence to which the children had been exposed, and that the success of the study depended on total honesty.

Measures

Parents completed the parent report version of the Checklist of Child Distress Symptoms (CCDS – Richters and Martinez 1990a), which was developed for this study from diagnostic criteria described in the *Diagnostic and Statistical Manual of Mental Disorders* (3rd ed, revised – American Psychiatric Association 1987). The CCDS questionnaire includes 28 symptom descriptions, each with a Likert scale response format for rating symptom presence on a 1–4 scale ranging from (1) never to (4) a lot of the time. Parents also completed the Child Behavior Checklist (CBCL), a widely used checklist of children's behavior problems for which a considerable body of reliability and validity data have been published (Achenbach and Edelbrock 1983). Finally, as described in detail elsewhere, parents completed the parent-report version of Survey of Children's Exposure to Community Violence concerning details of their children's exposure to violence in the community (Richters and Martinez 1992).

First- and second-grade children were assembled in small groups to participate in two age-appropriate interviews. The first was a cartoon-based interview of children's distress symptoms (*Levonn* – Richters, Martinez, and Valla 1990) based on the original work of Valla (1989) and modified to (1) depict the central character (*Dominique*) as an urban child (*Levonn*), (2) include depictions of symptoms associated with posttraumatic stress disorder not included in the original interview, (3) include a 2-3 sentence script with each carton, and (4) include a new response format for indicating frequency, consisting of thermometers filled with varying degrees of mercury.

Above each cartoon was a picture of three thermometers, each filled with a different level of mercury, labeled "never," "some of the time," and "a lot of the time," respectively. Prior to administration, children were taught how to use the thermometer response format correctly to indicate

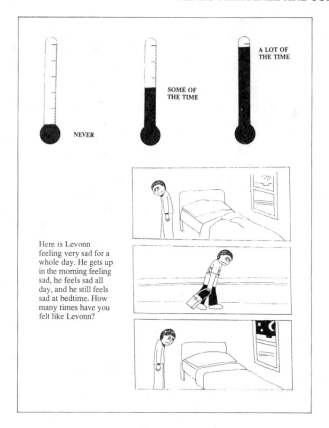

Figure 1.
Sample cartoon from *Levonn*, a distress symptom interview
for young children.

frequency. Next, each child was given a numbered set of the cartoon depictions; each cartoon was described orally from a script. Following each cartoon description, children were asked to circle a thermometer indicating how often they felt like *Levonn*. As detailed elsewhere, younger children also completed *Things I Have Seen and Heard*, a simply worded structured interview that assesses the frequency of children's exposure to violence and violence related themes (Richters and Martinez, 1992). One week text–retest data based on *Levonn* were collected from a random subsample of younger children. Reliability for the composite distress rating computed by summing across all symptom scores was high and significant, $r(22) = .81, p < .001$. Across the full sam-

ple of younger children, the composite symptom score based on *Levonn* was significantly related to parent-rated CBCL scores, $r(76) = .30, p < .01$, and to parent ratings of children's distress based on the CCDS, $r(76) = .32, p < .01$.

Children in grades 5 and 6 completed the self-report version of the Checklist of Child Distress Symptoms (CCDS) completed earlier by their parents about them. As described in the earlier report, they also completed the self-report version of the Survey of Children's Exposure to Community Violence concerning details of the frequency and context of their exposure to various forms of violence in the community (Richters and Saltzman 1990). Older children also completed the Child Depression Inventory (CDI), a widely used measure of children's self-reported depressive symptoms (Kovaks 1985). Children's composite symptom scores based on the CCDS were significantly related to their CDI scores, $r(37) = .49, p < .01$.

RESULTS

Sample Characteristics

Elsewhere we have shown that (1) families of younger and older children did not differ significantly on any of the major demographic characteristics assessed, (2) there were no significant differences in teacher-rated family violence or family stability between participating and non-participating families for either age group, (3) children of participating and nonparticipating families did not differ significantly on teacher ratings of classroom-based behavior problems or overall student progress, and (4) the study school, according to police statistics, was located in a moderately violent Ward of Washington, DC (Richters and Martinez 1992).

Distress Symptoms in Younger Children

First- and second-grade children's responses to the cartoon-based symptom interview were reduced initially to four scales, representing depression (10 items, Chronbach's $\alpha = .78$), anxiety/intrusive thoughts (14 items, Chronbach's $\alpha = .84$), and sleep problems (7 items, Chronbach's $\alpha = .71$). Girls reported significantly higher levels of depression, $t(75) = 1.66, p = .05$; anxiety/intrusive thoughts, $t(75) = 1.72$, $p < .05$; and sleep problems, $t(75) = 1.84$, $p < .05$, compared to boys. In contrast, boys reported slightly higher levels of impulsiveness than girls, although the difference was nonsignificant. Correlations among the scales (r values: .64–.85) were sufficiently high to justify combining them into a single index of children's distress symptoms.

The age-appropriate wording and response format of the young children's symptom interviews differed substantial-

ly from the symptom checklist completed by their parents, precluding direct comparisons of parents' and children's reports of absolute symptom levels. Parent–child agreement about the relative levels of children's symptoms was modest but significant across all children, $r(76) = .32, p < .01$. Whereas parent–child agreement was significant for boys, $r(38) = .41, p < .01$, it did not reach significance for girls, $r(38) = .19$, NS. This prompted us to examine differences between characteristics of the girls' and boys' families that might account for the absence of parent–daughter agreement. As expected, families of boys and girls did not differ significantly on any of the major demographic characteristics assessed. There was, however, a sizable and significant overall difference in the levels of severe within-family violence reported by parents of boys (mean = 1.63,) and girls (mean = 4.92), $t(70) = 2.43, p < .05$. Moreover, this difference was associated with a significantly wider range of within-family violence scores for families of boys (0 to 14) and girls (0 to 26). We therefore reexamined mother–daughter agreement about the daughters' distress symptoms within the more restricted range of within-family severe violence scores defined by the boys' families. Parent–daughter agreement for this subset of families was moderate and significant, $r(31) = .34, p < .05$, and did not differ significantly from agreement between boys and their parents. Given the relatively small number of families at the highest end of the severe within-family violence range, it was not possible to explore alternative models to account for the absence of parent–daughter agreement in the most violent families.

Violence exposure and distress symptoms. The associations between child-reported violence exposure and both child- and parent-reported symptoms are presented in Table 1. As indicated, children's reports of their victimization by violence in the community were significantly related to their overall self-ratings of distress symptoms, $r(31) = .28, p < .01$, and significantly more strongly to their spe-

Table 1

OLDER CHILDREN'S DISTRESS SYMPTOMS: COMPARISON
OF PARENTS' AND CHILDREN'S REPORT

Distress Symptom	Parents' Ratings (n = 35) Mean (SD)	Children's Ratings (n = 35) Mean (SD)	t	p
Trouble paying attention	2.75 (.96)	2.41 (.95)	1.53	NS
Daydreaming in class	2.38 (.95)	2.24 (.80)	.57	NS
Don't feel like doing fun things	2.05 (1.1)	2.36 (.96)	1.26	NS
Don't care about anything	1.73 (.80)	2.16 (1.09)	2.21	<.05
Worry about being safe	2.03 (1.18)	3.28 (.82)	4.88	<.001
Intrusive thoughts about upsetting events	1.78 (.90)	2.67 (.92)	3.96	<.001
Hard time getting/staying asleep	1.57 (.96)	2.43 (1.07)	3.22	<.01
Jumpy when hearing loud noises	1.88 (.98)	2.41 (.93)	2.18	<.05
Bad dreams/nightmares	1.70 (.85)	1.86 (.82)	.75	NS
Avoids upsetting situations	1.56 (.93)	2.50 (1.1)	4.07	<.001
Difficult time avoiding fear	1.61 (.90)	2.27 (.91)	3.22	<.01
Feel lonely	1.61 (.96)	2.22 (1.10)	2.25	<.05
Feel nervous, scared, upset	1.81 (.87)	2.32 (.74)	2.79	<.01
Easily bothered/upset	1.82 (.81)	2.24 (.86)	2.05	.05
Afraid might not live long	1.08 (.50)	1.75 (1.05)	3.28	<.01
Afraid might not have happy life	1.27 (.65)	1.67 (.97)	2.12	.05
Trouble remembering frightening events	1.34 (.59)	2.03 (.92)	4.21	<.001
Summary Scales				
Depression	1.66 (.48)	2.07 (.47)	3.42	<.01
Anxiety	1.88 (.46)	2.29 (.37)	3.79	<.01

cific ratings of fear while in school, $r(81) = .50$, $p < .01$ and at home, $r(81) = .43$, $p < .01$.

Children's reports of *witnessing* violence in the community were also associated with higher self-ratings of overall distress, $r(81) = .30$, $p < .01$, but not to fear at school, $r(81) = .07$, ns, or at home, $r(81) = .09$, ns. Similarly, children's ratings of how often they had seen guns or drugs in their homes were significantly associated with overall distress, $r(81) = .30$, $p < .01$, fear while at school, $r(81) = .36$, $p < .01$, and fear at home, $r(81) = .25$, $p < .01$. The relative contributions of the three forms of violence exposure to a composite index (a sum of the z scores for each measure) of children's distress symptoms were examined using a forward stepwise regression model. After controlling for the contribution of child-reported victimization to the prediction of children's distress symptoms, $r = .54$, $F(1, 77) = 31.09$, $p < .001$; adj $r^2 = .28$, neither of the other exposure variables entered the equation. Similar results were obtained when other predictors were entered into the equation first; the remaining variables and their interactions failed to make a significant incremental contribution to variance in children's distress symptoms beyond the variance accounted for by the initial exposure variable. None of the children's reports of exposure to violence were related significantly to parent-completed CBCL ratings.

To isolate the violence exposure variables most associated with high levels of distress symptoms, we compared children with the highest levels of self-reported distress (above the 75th percentile) with the remaining children on each of the child-reported violence exposure variables. Children experiencing the highest levels of distress were more likely to report having been threatened with a knife, $r(82) = 2.59$, $p = .01$, and having witnessed someone being stabbed, $t(82) = 2.30$, $p < .01$, drugs in the home, $t(82) = 2.60$, $p < .01$, and guns in the home, $t(82) = 2.38$, $p < .01$.

Mediators of exposure–distress. In a series of exploratory analyses we tested for demographic mediators of the link between children's violence exposure and distress symptoms. Most demographic factors were unrelated to the exposure–distress association. There was one exception. The exposure–distress link was significantly stronger for children of parents who had not graduated high school, $r(15) = .65$, $p < .01$, than for children of parents who had graduated high school, $r(60) = .37$, $p < .01$.[2] Although there was also a trend for girls to come from homes with less-educated parents, $\chi^2(1) = 2.80$, $p = .09$, their reports of violence exposure were no more likely to be associated with distress symptoms than those of boys, $r(38) = .39$ vs. $r(37) = .44$, respectively, $p < .01$ in each case. Nor is it the case that the children of less educated parents were more likely to misunderstand the questions and/or indiscriminately rate all of their responses high; the absolute levels of violence exposure and distress symptoms they reported did not differ significantly from the reports of children with better educated parents, $t(73) = .51$ and $.57$, respectively. Although the association between violence exposure and distress symptoms was not significantly mediated by other demographic factors we examined, it is nonetheless worth noting that families with less-educated parents were also characterized by higher levels of unemployment, $t(62) = 5.14$, $p < .001$, public assistance, $t(59) = 4.10$, $p < .001$, and trends toward a higher level of mother absence, $t(63) = 1.46$, $p = .07$ and father absence, $t(63) = 1.31$, $p = .12$. Due to distributional and sample size restrictions, however, it is impossible to determine the extent to which these variables, alone or in combination, contributed to the exposure–distress association in younger children.

---

[2]Two bivariate outliers with extremely high exposure scores and extremely low distress scores were excluded from these analyses.

Distress Symptoms in Older Children

Fifth- and sixth-grade children's ratings of their distress symptoms on the CCDS were combined initially into two correlated scales of moderately high reliability: depression ($\alpha = .71$) and anxiety ($\alpha = .72$); $r(37) = .64$, $p < .001$. Identical analyses were conducted on the parent-report version of the CCDS, again yielding correlated scales for depression ($\alpha = .75$) and anxiety ($\alpha = .70$), $r(51) = .80$, $p < .001$.

Analyses of variance revealed no significant differences between boys' and girls' depression and anxiety levels according to either parents' or children's own reports. As indicated in Table 1, children overall reported significantly higher levels of depression, $t(34) = 3.42$, $p < .01$, and anxiety, $t(34) = 3.79$, $p < .01$, symptoms than their parents reported about them. In light of the relatively high correlations between depression and anxiety for both children's and parents' reports, these scales were combined for each informant, yielding separate indices of children's distress based on parent and child reports.

For descriptive purposes, child–parent comparisons for individual distress symptoms are also presented in Table 1. As indicated, children reported significantly higher levels of distress than their parents reported about them in response to 22 (72%) of the 28 symptoms probed. These comparisons do not, however, adequately convey the extent to which parents underestimated the distress symptoms of their older children. For example, 49% of the parents reported that their children never worried about being safe, whereas *none* of their children said they never worried, $\chi^2(1) = 48.57$, $p < .001$; in contrast, only 16% of the parents reported that their children worried about being safe a lot of the time, compared to 50% of their children, $\chi^2(1) = 18.63$, $p < .001$. Similarly, 53% of the parents reported that their children were never bothered by intrusive thoughts about upsetting events, compared to only 8% of their children, $\chi^2(1) = 33.95$, $p < .001$. On the other end of the continuum, 22% of the children reported being bothered by such intrusive thoughts, compared to *none* of their parents, $\chi^2(1)$ = 16.96, $p < .001$. Parents also significantly underestimated the extent to which their older children suffered problems either getting or staying asleep at night. Whereas only 27% of the parents reported that their children ever suffered from sleeping problems, 70% of their children reported sleeping problems at least some of the time, $\chi^2(1) = 25.31$, $p < .001$.

Parent–child agreement. Consistent with our earlier report showing poor parent–daughter agreement about violence exposure (Richters and Martinez 1993), agreement between parents and daughters about their daughters' distress symptoms was low and nonsignificant, $r(17) = .06$. In contrast, agreement between parents and their sons was moderately high *and negative*, $r(18) = -.56$, $p < .01$ (not attributable to outliers). Boys who rated themselves low in distress despite being rated high by their parents reported community violence exposure levels quite similar to the levels reported by other boys, $t(16) = .59$, ns, suggesting that they did not have a general tendency to withhold or underreport information. Moreover, although parents' CBCL-based anxiety ratings were strongly related to their ratings of their sons' anxiety on the CCDS distress questionnaire, $r(18) = .63$, $p < .01$, their association with mother-rated antisocial behavior was low and nonsignificant, $r(21) = .22$, ns. Thus, antisocial behavior was not a significant correlate of mother-rated anxiety in the boys. But boys who rated themselves low in distress despite being rated as high in distress by their parents were significantly more likely to have been rated by their parents as boastful and/or bragging on the CBCL (item 7) than boys who agreed with their parents about high distress, $t(9) = 4.43$, $p < .001$. They were also rated as significantly more boastful/bragging than all other boys combined, $t(17) = 2.79$, $p < .01$. The partial correlation between parents' and sons' ratings of the sons' distress levels while controlling for their bragging/boasting scores was reduced to a nonsig-

nificant though still negative level, $r(15) = -.34$, ns.

Violence exposure and distress symptoms. As indicated in Table 2, older children's reports of victimization by and witnessing violence in the community involving persons known to them (family, friends, acquaintances) were significantly related to their self-reports of distress and depression (r .35–.42, p's < .05). The combined score reflecting victimization by and witnessing violence in the community involving those familiar to the children was more strongly associated with self-reported distress symptoms, $r(37) = .48$, $p < .01$. Children's reports of victimization by and witnessing violence involving strangers were not, however, related to their self-reports of distress or depression. Also, children's reports of violence (slapping, hitting, punching) within the home were significantly correlated with their reports of distress symptoms, $r(37) = .33$, $p < .05$.

The contributions of community and within-family violence exposure to the older children's reports of distress symptoms were examined using hierarchical multiple regression models. Results indicate that the significant community violence exposure correlates shared overlapping variance with distress symptoms. Once any of these variables was entered into the regression model as a predictor of distress symptoms, none of the remaining variables contributed significantly to the equation.

Exploratory analyses revealed that the association between violence exposure and distress symptoms based on children's reports was mediated by maternal education, such that exposure was more strongly predictive of distress symptoms in children of parents with little or no education, $r(10) = .64$, $p < .05$, than in children of parents who had graduated high school, $r(25) = .29$, ns. Thus, these results parallel the findings reported above for younger children.

To isolate the violence exposure variables most associated with high levels of

Table 2
SYMPTOM CORRELATES OF CHILDREN'S VIOLENCE EXPOSURE

Children's Symptoms

Older Children's Violence Exposure[a]	Mother CBCL (n = 36)	Mother-Rated Distress (n = 35)	Child-Rated Distress (n = 37)	Child-Rated CDI (n = 37)		
Community violence victimization[b]	.13/.09	.06/.05	.37*/.08	.42**/.01		
Community violence witnessed[c]	.03/−.20	.01/−.22	.39*/−.05	.35*/.01		
Home violence witnessed[d]	.04	.11	.33*	.24		

Younger Children's Violence Exposure	Mother CBCL (n = 77)	Mother-Rated Distress (n = 76)	Child-Rated Distress (n = 84)		Child-Rated Fear at School (n = 82)	Child-Rated Fear at Home (n = 81)
Community violence victimization[b]	.10	.12	.28**		.50**	.43**
Community violence witnessed[c]	−.04	−.02	.30**		.07	.09
Witnessed guns/drugs in home[d]	.13	.13	.30**		.36**	.25*

[a]Correlations based on violence involving family, friends, and aquaintances appear before the slash; those based on violence involving strangers appears after the slash.
[b]Frequency of exposure across all forms of victimization.
[c]Frequency of exposure across all forms of witnessing slapping, hitting, and/or punching in the home.
[d]Sum of frequency of witnessing guns and/or drugs in the home.
*$p < .05$.
**$p < .01$.

distress symptoms, we compared children with the highest levels of self-reported distress (75th percentile and above) with those below the 75th percentile on each of the violence exposure variables. Children in the high-distress group were more likely than other children to have witnessed drug deals, $t(35) = 2.49, p < .01$; people being arrested, $t(34) = 2.02, p < .05$; someone being slapped, punched, or hit by a family member, $t(35) = 3.29, p < .01$; and someone carrying an illegal weapon, $t(35) = 2.17, p < .05$.

DISCUSSION

The data from this study indicate that violence exposure was associated with distress symptoms in both older and younger children. For children in both groups, victimization by violence in the community and witnessing violence or violence-related themes in both the community and at home were reliably related to greater levels of distress symptoms. Although the majority of violence experienced by the children took place outside their homes, reports from the older children indicate that the majority of those events involved persons familiar to the children, including family members, friends, and acquaintances. Moreover, older children's reports of distress symptoms and depression were significantly associated *only* with violence involving persons known to them. It was also the case that younger children with the highest levels of self-reported distress symptoms were significantly more likely than other children to report having seen guns and drugs in their homes. Thus, we know from the present data that reports of victimization by and witnessing violence in the community as well as witnessing themes of violence in the home is already associated with classic distress symptoms among very young children. Parents from the most violent homes were significantly less likely to agree with their children about their children's distress symptoms. To the extent that this reflects

a genuine lack of parental awareness of the children's symptoms, it may place their children at an additional disadvantage for coping.

An equally striking finding was the extent to which parents underestimated levels of distress their children were experiencing. Certainly, the fact that parents tend to underestimate their children's feelings and emotions is a well-replicated finding in the child psychopathology literature (Achenbach, McConaughy, and Howell 1987; Herjanic and Reich 1982; Kashani, Orvaschel, Burk, and Reid 1985), albeit one with largely unknown implications for children's social–emotional development. But this phenomenon may take on even added significance when the children's symptoms are associated with objectively dangerous experiences. Children whose parents are unaware of their distress symptoms may be at heightened risk for developing maladaptive coping responses, and for overgeneralizing initially adaptive distress reactions to situations and contexts in which those responses are maladaptive. Parents who are unaware of their children's distress may miss important opportunities to offer consul and to help their children cope with violence they have already experienced as well as develop strategies for avoiding violent situations in the future.

These parent–child discrepancies also underscore the need for researchers to interview children directly in attempts to assess their reactions to violent events. Children as young as age 6 in this study were able and quite willing to discuss their feelings and concerns about violence and distress when given the opportunity, yielding information that was unavailable from their parents' reports. In the case of older children, there was evidence that boys rated by their parents as high on anxiety tended to deny those symptoms, and this denial was significantly associated with higher scores on bragging and boasting. This pattern, which was not present in the younger boys, may signal for a subset of boys a developmental shift toward bravado and the denial of anxieties and fears that are nonetheless recognized by their parents. The conditions under which this process develops and its implications for development – particularly among children living in dangerous environments – deserve careful attention in future longitudinal designs. Moreover, the fact that violence exposure was more strongly related to distress symptoms in both younger and older children from households with less-educated parents suggests that these children may be at particularly high risk for developing maladaptive responses to violence exposure. Collectively, these data highlight the need for intervention programs in high-risk neighborhoods that can employ methods for helping children talk about their distress, and for helping parents to recognize and deal with symptoms of distress in their children.

In light of the cross-sectional nature of this study, it is impossible to examine the extent to which children's reported symptoms preceded and perhaps even gave rise to, rather than followed, their exposure to violence. One can easily imagine children who, for a variety of reasons associated with maladjustment, find themselves in situations in which they are exposed to higher than average rates of violence. For these children, it may be maladjustment that gives rise to violence exposure. It is also possible that some children, for reasons other than violence exposure, are suffering from symptoms of distress, and for that reason have a heightened sensitivity to actual as well as misperceived violence in their environments. Each of these possibilities deserves careful attention in subsequent research and can be most easily studied using short-term longitudinal designs.

Finally, our focus in this report on children's distress symptoms associated with violence exposure should not obscure the fact that we know very little about either the immediate or long-term implications of these symptoms. To be sure, some symptoms can be seen as normal reactions to abnormal events. Certain types of fear, anxiety, intrusive thoughts, and even depression can serve adaptive functions in an objectively dangerous environment, particularly when they signal heightened vigilance and healthy emotional reactions to loss and pain. But just as clearly they can signal maladaptive reactions with long-term negative consequences for normal social, emotional, and cognitive development. This can even happen when initially adaptive responses become entrenched, resistant to change, and overgeneralized to situations in which they are maladaptive. In the present study, parent ratings of children's behavior problems were *not* significantly associated with either parent- or child-reported violence exposure. Given the pattern of disparities between parent and child reports, however, this should not be interpreted as evidence that distress symptoms are unrelated to children's behavior problems. An important task for future research will be to develop assessment strategies for discriminating more effectively between adaptive and maladaptive reactions to violence, and for detecting maladaptive response patterns before they become pathological. Obviously, the pursuit of these issues will also require sensitive strategies for combining data from multiple informants to assess children's distress symptoms and role-functioning impairments.

Beyond distress symptoms per se, much remains to be learned about the impact of chronic violence exposure. Domains that warrant consideration include children's ability to experience and modulate arousal; their images of themselves; their beliefs in a just and benevolent world; their beliefs about the likelihood of surviving into adulthood; their willingness to form and maintain affective relationships with parents, siblings, and peers who may not survive the violence; the value they place on human life; their sense of morality; and a range of other topics central to normal/adaptive development.

REFERENCES

ACHENBACH, T. M. and EDELBROCK, C. S. *Manual for the Child Behavior Checklist and Revised Behavior Profile*. University of Vermont Department of Psychiatry, 1983.

ACHENBACH, T. M., MCCONAUGHY, S., and HOWELL, C. T. Child/adolescent behavioral and emotional problems: Implications of cross-informant correlations for situational specificity. *Psychological Bulletin* (1987) 101:213–22.

AMERICAN PSYCHIATRIC ASSOCIATION *Diagnostic and Statistical Manual of Mental Disorders*, 3rd ed., rev. American Psychiatric Association, 1987.

BODMAN, F. War conditions and the mental health of the child. *British Medical Journal* (1941) 2(Part 2):286–88.

BREZNITZ, S., ed. *Stress in Israel*. Van Nostrand Reinhold, 1983.

BROWN, G. W., HARRIS, T. O., and BIFULCO, A. Long-term effects of early loss of a parent. In M. Rutter, C. E. Izard, and P. B. Read, eds., *Depression in Young People: Developmental and Clinical Perspectives*. Guilford Press, 1986.

BURKE, J. D., BORUS, J. F., BURNS, B. J., MILSTEIN, K. H., and BEASLEY, M. C. Changes in children's behavior after a natural disaster. *American Journal of Psychiatry*, (1982) 139:1010–14.

CICCHETTI, D., and RIZLEY, R. Developmental perspectives on the etiology, intergenerational transmission and sequela of child maltreatment. In R. Rizley and D. Cicchetti, eds. *New Directions of Child Development* (pp. 31–56). Josey-Bass, 1981.

CHRISTOFEL, K. K. Violent death and injury in US children and adolescents. *American Journal of Disease Control* (1990) 144:697–706.

COMPAS, B. Stress and life events during childhood and adolescence. *Clinical Psychology Review* (1987) 7:275–302.

EMERY, R. E. Interparental conflict and the children of discord and divorce. *Psychological Bulletin* (1982) 92:310–30.

FREUD, A., and BURLINGHAM, D. T. *Children and War*. London: Medical War Books, 1982.

GALANTE, R., and FOA, D. An epidemiological study of psychic trauma and treatment effectiveness for children after a natural disaster. *Journal of the American Academy of Child Psychiatry* (1986) 25:357–63.

GARMEZY, N. Children under severe stress: Critique and commentary. *Journal of the American Academy of Child Psychiatry* (1986) 25:384–92.

GARMEZY, N., and RUTTER, M. Acute reactions to stress. In M. Rutter and L. Hersov, eds., *Child and Adolescent Psychiatry: Modern Approaches*, 2nd ed. (pp. 152–176). Blackwell Scientific Publications, 1985.

GLOVER, E. Notes on the psychological effects of war conditions on the civilian population. Part III: The blitz. *International Journal of Psychoanalysis*, (1942) 29(Part 1):17–37.

HANDFORD, H. A., MAYES, S. D., MATTISON, R. E.,

HUMPHREY, F. J., BAGNATO, S., BIXLER, E. O., and KALES, J. D. Child and parent reactions to the Three Mile Island nuclear accident. *Journal of the American Academy of Child Psychiatry* (1986) 25:346–56.

HERJANIC, B., and REICH, W. Development of a structured psychiatric interview for children: Agreement between child and parent on individual symptoms. *Journal of Abnormal Child Psychology* (1982) 10:307–24.

JOHN, E. M. A study of the effects of evacuation and air raids on children of pre-school age. *British Journal of Educational Psychology* (1941) 11:173–82.

KASHANI, J. H., ORVASCHEL, H., BURK, J. P., and REID, J. C. Informant variance: The issue of parent–child agreement. *Journal of the American Academy of Child Psychiatry* (1985) 24:437–41.

KOVAKS, M. The Children's Depression Inventory. *Psychopharmacology Bulletin* (1985) 21:995–98.

KINZIE, J. D., SACK, W. H., ANGELL, R. H., MANSON, S., and RATH, B. The psychiatric effects of massive trauma on Cambodian children: I. The children. *Journal of the American Academy of Child Psychiatry* (1986) 25:370–76.

LACY, G. N. Observations on Aberfan. *Journal of Psychosomatic Research* (1972) 16:257–60.

LEBOVICI, S. Observations on children who have witnessed the violent death of one of their parents: A contribution to the study of traumatization. *International Review of Psychoanalysis* (1974) 1:117–23.

LYONS, H. A. The psychological effects of the civil disturbance on children. *Northern Teacher* (1973) (Winter):35–38.

LYONS, H. A. Civil violence – The psychological aspects. *Journal of Psychosomatic Research* (1979) 23:373–93.

MCAULEY, R., and TROY, M. The impact of urban conflict and violence on children referred to a child psychiatry clinic. In J. Harbison, ed., *Children of the Troubles* (pp. 33–43). Belfast: Stranmillis College, 1983.

MCWHIRTER, L. Yoked by violence together: Stress and coping in children in Northern Ireland. *Community Care* (1982) (Nov. 4):14–17.

MCWHIRTER, L. Growing up in Northern Ireland: From "aggression" to the "troubles." In A. P. Goldstein and M. H. Segall, eds., *Aggression in Global Perspective* (pp. 367–400). Pergamon Press, 1983.

MCWHIRTER, L., and TREW, K. Children in Northern Ireland: A lost generation? In E. J. Anthony and C. Chiland, eds., *The Child in His Family. Children in Turmoil: Tomorrow's Children*, Vol 7 (pp. 69–82). Wiley Interscience, 1981.

MILGRAM, N. A. War-related stress in Israeli children and youth. In L. Goldberger and S. Breznitz, eds. *Handbook of Stress: Theoretical and Clinical Aspects* (pp. 656–76). Free Press, 1982.

MILGRAM, R. M., and MILGRAM, N. A. The effect of

the Yom Kippur war on anxiety level in Israeli children. *Journal of Psychology* (1976) 94:107–13.

PUBLIC HEALTH SERVICE. *Healthy People 2000: National Health Promotion and Disease Prevention Objectives.* U.S. Department of Health and Human Services, 1990.

PYNOOS, R. S., FREDERICK, C., NADER, K., ARROYO, W., STEINBERGH, A., ETH, S., NUNEZ, F., and FAIRBANKS, L. Life threat and posttraumatic stress in school-age children. *Archives of General Psychiatry* (1987) 44:1057–63.

RICHTERS, J. E., and MARTINEZ, P. *Checklist of Child Distress Symptoms: Parent Report.* National Institute of Mental Health, 1990a.

RICHTERS, J. E., MARTINEZ, P., and VALLA, J.-P. *Levonn: A Cartoon-Based Structured Interview for Assessing Young Children's Distress Symptoms.* National Institute of Mental Health, 1990b.

RICHTERS, J. E., and MARTINEZ, P. The NIMH community violence project: I. Children as victims of and witnesses to violence. *Psychiatry* (1993) 56:7–21.

RICHTERS, J. E., and SALTZMAN, W. *Survey of Children's Exposure to Community Violence: Parent Report.* National Institute of Mental Health, 1990.

ROSENBLATT, R. *Children of War.* Anchor Press/Doubleday, 1983.

SACK, W. H., AANGELL, R. H., KINZIE, J. D., and RATH, B. The psychiatric effects of massive trauma on Cambodian children: II. The family, the home, and the school. *Journal of the American Academy of Child Psychiatry* (1986) 25:377–83.

SATTLER, J. M. Racial "experimenter effects" in experimentation, testing, interviewing, and psychotherapy. *Psychological Bulletin* (1970) 73:137–60.

SILBER, E., PERRY, and BLOCH, D. (1958). Patterns of parent–child interaction in a disaster. *Psychiatry* (1958) 21:159–67.

TERR, L. C. Children of Chowchilla: A study of psychic trauma. *Psychoanalytic Study of the Child* (1979) 34:552–623.

TERR, L. C. Forbidden games: Post-traumatic child's play. *Journal of American Academy of Child Psychiatry* (1981) 20:741–60.

TERR, L. C. Chowchilla revisited: The effects of psychic trauma four years after a school-bus kidnapping. *American Journal of Psychiatry* (1983) 140:1543–50.

VALLA, J.-P. *Dominique: A Cartoon Interview for Assessing Young Children's Psychiatric Symptoms.* University of Montreal, 1989.

WATT, N. F., ANTHONY, E. J., WYNNE, L. C., and ROLF, J. E., eds. *Children at Risk for Schizophrenia: A Longitudinal Perspective.* Cambridge University Press, 1984.

ZIV, A., and ISRAEL, R. Effects of bombardment on the manifest anxiety level of children living in the kibbutzim. *Journal of Consulting and Clinical Psychology* (1973) 40:287–91.

Chronic Community Violence: What Is Happening to Our Children?

Joy D. Osofsky, Sarah Wewers, Della M. Hann, and Ana C. Fick

CHRONIC violence is a growing problem in our society today as evidenced, among other factors, by the ever-increasing murder rate in many of our large urban centers in the United States. Emphasis has begun to be placed on chronic violence, causes that may contribute to it, and the impact of this violence on cities and the country at large. While concern has been expressed, we still have not addressed adequately, nor do we fully understand, the effects on the children who must grow up in environments where they are repeatedly being exposed to significant levels of violence.

In the present paper, focus is placed on elementary schoolchildren growing up in and around the Desire/Florida Housing development in New Orleans, Louisiana, one of the largest housing development units in the United States. Not only is this housing development one of the largest, but the area in and around it (District 5) ranks among the highest for violence in the city (see Figure 1). In 1989, in the 12.4 square miles of the city in which this project is located, there were 72 murders, 91 rapes, 1521 assaults, and 1114 armed robberies. The incidence of other less violent crimes was 8944, combining to a total of 11,742 reported crimes for a population of about 121,300. The numbers and percentage of violent crimes in this area continued to increase in 1990, with 84 murders being reported for the year.

What is the experience of families and children who are living in such environments? How can we even hope to socialize children to grow up to be humane, compassionate, nurturant, and loving?

Although all of the expected outcomes from children's exposure to chronic violence cannot be determined at this time, we know that communities are affected greatly by these events. The literature related to isolated exposure to traumatic violent events such as sniper attacks or random shootings and outcomes for children may be instructive, although limited, when attempting to apply findings to children exposed to chronic urban violence. Evaluating stress symptoms experienced by children exposed to acute trauma may help us understand the potential problems that may occur for children living under conditions of chronic violence. Frederick (1985), discussing children who were traumatized by different types of catastrophic situations such as sniper attacks, unexpected gunfire, or the death of someone close to them, reported fears of recur-

Joy D. Osofsky, Sarah Wewers, Della M. Hann, and Ana C. Fick are with the Louisiana State University Medical Center.

This research was supported by grants from the Early Childhood Transition Network of the John D. and Catherine T. MacArthur Foundation and by the Institute of Mental Hygiene of New Orleans. Special appreciation is given to the Lockett Elementary School and the parents for their cooperation with this project.

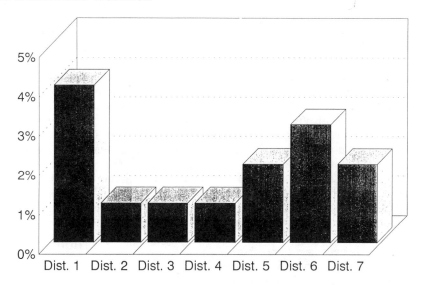

Figure 1.
Proportion of violent crimes, by district: New Orleans, 1989.

rence, continuing concerns about security, anger, and preoccupations about revenge, among other problems.

Pynoos et al. (1987), using the Post-Traumatic Stress Disorder (PTSD) Index, studied both the acute and chronic reactions of 159 elementary schoolchildren sampled after a sniper attack on their school playground. They found significant relationships between proximity to the violence, that is, violence exposure, and type and number of PTSD symptoms. Differences were found between children exposed to this particular sniper event and those who were exposed to chronic violence in their neighborhoods but not this specific event, suggesting that acute traumatic events may increase the incidence of PTSD symptoms even when children live in high-violence areas. Pynoos and Nader (1989), in another study, reported that children who witness injury to others and hear their cries for help may be especially vulnerable to reexperience the violent event. This reexperiencing occurs commonly as traumatic dreams, which include fears of recurrence or other forms of violence or life threat. Others (Kramer et al. 1984) have reported that fears of trau-

matic dreams may lead to sleep disturbances or fear of sleeping alone. Furthermore, in play, children may repeat the traumatic themes, particularly those of fear and/or aggression (Terr 1990).

Clinical descriptive studies done following sniper attacks (Pynoos and Nader 1989) or other traumatic events such as the experience of 26 children who were kidnapped from their school bus and buried alive (Terr 1990) have reported follow-up symptoms of reduced involvement with the external world resulting in constricted affect, fewer interests, and feelings of estrangement. Another symptom complex that has been observed in children is avoidance of traumatic reminders of the event and/or memory impairment, which can lead to phobic behavior or constriction in cognition and daily activities. These studies of symptoms following isolated traumatic events are different but may be helpful in attempting to understand reactions and outcomes for children living in situations of chronic violence. In situations where children live with daily incidents of violence, it could be expected that such reactions might severely constrict their lives both at school and in their other activities. Even television may be avoided for fear of television violence as a traumatic reminder of the event (Kristal 1982).

Another area of concern for children who are exposed to chronic violence is loss and grief reactions. Young children living in high-crime and high-violence areas must deal with death more frequently and at younger ages than other children. Pynoos et al. (1987) followed 262 children 1 year after a sniper attack on their school playground. They found a linear relationship between familiarity with the deceased schoolmate and grief responses. Often the grief reactions that children experience seem to be confusing and frightening. They frequently do not understand the kinds of fantasies and nightmares that they experience about the dead person. They are reluctant to talk with others about their experience and, thus, often receive little support. These reactions have been observed in children exposed to only one traumatic event. For those exposed to repeated traumas, even more confusion and negative outcomes can be expected. Further, the parents of these children may have difficulty dealing with their own grief and providing their children with needed support.

While it is not possible to generalize from the findings of studies on reactions to isolated traumatic events to those of children living with chronic violence, these studies may be instructive in describing the range and variety of possible responses. Such related studies can help us learn more about some of stress responses that might be expected in situations with chronic violence.

Our current study resulted from a joint effort between colleagues in Washington, DC, and New Orleans. A group of researcher/clinicians in Washington, DC (Martinez and Richters 1993; Richters and Martinez 1993) initiated a project to study the effects of exposure to chronic community violence on children in several areas in the District of Columbia. Based on mutual concerns about the effects of vi-

olence on children, we selected an elementary school in New Orleans that was in a very violent area (as already described) and where administrators and teachers were willing to cooperate with us in carrying out a survey of the violence exposure of the children. Although the incidence of violent crime in the area was known and assumptions were made about children's exposure, documentation of the extent of the problem was needed. This documentation is considered to be very important as a first step toward developing broader research and intervention efforts.

METHODS

Subjects

The design for the New Orleans study was developed collaboratively with colleagues in Washington, DC (Martinez and Richters 1993; Richters and Martinez 1993). The objective of the study was to learn more about the amount and kinds of violence that children are exposed to as a first step in attempting to evaluate the effects on children. In order to accomplish this objective, our goal was to survey a group of elementary school children in relation to their violence exposure and to evaluate, through mothers' reports, related stress symptoms and behavior problems. Recruitment of subjects was done with the help of the principal and staff–parent facilitator at one of the elementary schools serving the Desire/Florida Housing development area. The staff–parent facilitator composed a letter explaining the project, gave it to the teachers of fifth-grade students, and requested that they send it home to the parents. The mothers were told that we were trying to learn more about the effects of violence exposure on children and how parents deal with this situation. We told them further that by gathering more information about children's violence exposure, we would be able to develop more effective programs for these children. Fifty-three of the possible 83 mothers (64%) agreed to participate, and appointments were arranged and consent forms signed. It was not possible to interview all of the 83 mothers of fifth graders for the following reasons. Eleven mothers had agreed to be interviewed but did not come for their appointments. Three of the mothers had more than one child in the fifth grade. It was not possible to make appointments with the other mothers due to work schedules, inability to reach them, and transportation problems. According to the school administrators, there was no reason to believe that the group that was sampled was not representative of the total group of mothers of fifth graders in that school. The demographics for the sample are presented in Table 1.

Most of the families were single parent families of lower socioeconomic status. All were of Afro-American background. Of some interest, 48% of the mothers had become mothers as teenagers. The children ranged in age from 9 to 12 years.

Procedures

Mothers were interviewed and assessed using structured measures to evaluate their childrens' exposure to community violence as well as problematic and stressful behaviors that they had observed in them. In both administering and analyzing the data, an effort was made to consider separately family conflict and violence, and community violence. The measures that were used included the following:

1. Survey of Exposure to Community Violence – Parent Report Version: The Survey of Exposure to Community Violence (Richters and Saltzman 1990) was administered to the mothers as a structured interview. The survey evaluates exposure to severe violence (shootings, stabbings, and rapes), less severe violence (beatings and chasings), and moderately severe violence (threats, accidents, drug deals, and arrests). The survey included question sets that asked mothers to report their child's exposure to these violent incidents in terms of the following domains: (1) the presence/absence of that form of exposure (hearing about, witnessing, or victimization); (2) the frequency of the exposure; (3) the location of the incident (e.g., near home or school); and (4) the degree of familiarity with the victim or perpetrator of the incident. Additional question sets were asked regarding the witnessing and hearing about suicides, killings, woundings, dead bodies, and use of weapons.

2. Survey of Children's Stress Symptoms – Parent Report: The Survey of Children's Stress Symptoms (Richters 1990) is a measure developed for this study by the Washington, DC, group. It consists of a 28-item scale evaluating child behaviors

Table 1

DEMOGRAPHIC INFORMATION (*n* = 53)

Biological mother completed questionnaires	92.2%
Education less than high school	52.8%
Yearly income less than $12,000	86.8%
Welfare reliance: complete or most	60.4%
Marital status	
Married to father of child	13.7%
Separated from father of child	17.6%
Single/never married	41.2%
Single/divorced	23.5%
Single/widowed	2.0%
Mother began parenting before age 20	48.0%
Time child lives with biological parents	
Mother: most or all the time	84.9%
Father: most or all the time	18.9%

that are indicative of stress. Examples of child behaviors included in the survey are worries about safety, difficulties in sleeping, recurrence of upsetting thoughts, and feelings of loneliness and upset. Parents indicate the extent to which they have observed these behaviors in their children on a scale of: (1) never occur, (2) seldom occur, (3) occur once in a while, or (4) occur a lot of the time. The 28 items are summed to provide an indication of the degree to which parents observed stress behaviors in their children.

3. Conflict Tactics Scale: The Conflict Tactics Scale (Straus 1979) is a widely used scale designed to measure intrafamily conflict and violence. The scale consists of 19 items reflecting different means by which interpersonal conflict can be settled. Each item is rated according to the frequency of occurrence over the last year on a scale of 0, never occurred, to 6, occurred twice or more a month. The values for three items (throwing something, pushing/shoving someone, and slapping someone) were summed to form an index of minor family conflict. A severe family conflict index was formed in a similar manner by summing the values for five items (hitting with fist, hitting with object, beating someone, threatening with a weapon, using a weapon).

4. Child Behavior Checklist (CBCL): The Child Behavior Checklist (Achenbach and Edelbrock 1981) is a scale measuring behavior problems. Parents indicate whether behavioral descriptions are (0) not true at all, (1) somewhat true, (2) or very true of their child. The form of the CBCL used for this study is designed for children ages 4–16 and consists of 118 items. This scale yields a Total, an Internalizing, and an Externalizing score, all of which have been related to the other measures.

RESULTS

In order to parallel the analyses of the Washington, DC, data (see Richters and Martinez 1993) and aid in the comparabil-

ity of the two data sets, attention was focused on exploring the first domain of questions on the violence survey, the presence/absence of different forms of exposure to violent incidents. Forms of exposure were examined first in relation to individual types of violent incidents, for example, hearing about a shooting, witnessing a shooting, and being victimized by a shooting. In addition, summary variables concerning form of exposure were computed across the severe, less severe, and moderately severe violence categories. These summary variables reflected the number of violent categories to which the child had been exposed. For example, the witnessing of severe violence summary variable was calculated by summing the presence (score = 1) of witnessing a shooting, stabbing, or rape. Scores on the witnessing severe violence variable could range from a low of 0, indicating witnessing of no severe violence, to a high of 3, indicating witnessing of all three severe violence categories. Summary variables were computed for each form of violence exposure (hearing about, witnessing, and victimization) in terms of severe, less severe, and moderately severe violence categories, resulting in nine summary variables.

The summary variables were further combined to provide overall indices of form of exposure to violence. Overall victimization indicated the sum of the severe, less severe, and moderately severe victimization summary variables. The overall witnessing and overall hearing about clusters were computed in the same manner resulting in three overall cluster variables of form of exposure to violence.

The results from the Survey of Exposure to Community Violence showed that children living in this very violent area of the city were exposed to high levels of violence.

As can be seen in Table 2, almost the entire group had heard about some form of a violent episode, 91% had witnessed violence, and over half had been victims of some form of violence. Twenty-six percent of the sample had witnessed a shooting and 19% had witnessed a stabbing. Three

Table 2

PREVALENCE OF EXPOSURE TO DIFFERENT LEVELS OF VIOLENCE AND OCCURRENCE OF SPECIFIC VIOLENCE CATEGORIES

	Heard	Witness	Victim
Level of Violence			
Severe	79.2	37.7	5.7
Less severe	77.4	71.7	28.3
Moderate	96.2	86.7	33.9
Total	98.1	90.6	50.9
Violence Category			
Shooting	73.6	26.4	0.0
Stabbing	47.2	18.9	1.9 (n = 1)
Rape	34.0	3.8	3.8 (n = 2)
Weapons used	69.8	71.7	
Dead bodies	64.2	39.6	
Woundings	60.4	49.1	
Killings	75.5	5.7	
Suicides	26.4	1.9	

children had experienced personally the most severe forms of victimization, stabbing or rape. In addition to exposure to the various forms of violence, 40% of the parents reported that their children had seen a dead body, 72% had seen weapons being used, and 49% had seen someone who was wounded. The reports of having heard about these violent incidents were much higher.

The results of the survey data also showed strong and significant relationships between exposure to community violence (Survey of Exposure to Community Violence), the incidence of family violence (Conflict Tactics Scale), and the overall stress symptoms observed in the children (Survey of Stress Scale) (see Table 3).

There were significant relationships between hearing about and witnessing community violence and reports of stress symptoms in the children ($r = .48$ and $r = .42$, respectively). In addition, children's stress symptoms were highly related to the degree of severe family conflict ($r = .61$). In order to test for the effectiveness of multiple variables in predicting child stress symptoms, a stepwise multiple regression was performed. The child stress index was used as the criterion variable; and indices of community and family violence, as predictors. This

analysis indicated that three variables, family severe conflict ($r = .56$), witnessing of severe violence ($r = .35$), and hearing about violence ($r = .32$) accounted for 53% of the variance in reports of child stress symptoms ($R = .73$, $F = 17.33$, $p < .001$).

Table 4 presents a more detailed analysis of the relationships between community violence and family conflict. As can

Table 3

CORRELATIONS BETWEEN STRESS SYMPTOMS, COMMUNITY VIOLENCE, AND FAMILY CONFLICT

	Stress Symptoms
Community Violence	
Victimization	.21
Witnessing	.42***
Severe	.51***
Less severe	.29*
Moderate	.35**
Hearing about	.48***
Severe	.34*
Less severe	.31*
Moderate	.32*
Family Conflict Resolution	
Minor	.39***
Severe	.61***

*$p < .05$, **$p < .01$, ***$p < .005$ (based on two-tailed tests).

Table 4

RELATIONSHIPS BETWEEN MEASURES OF FAMILY
CONFLICT AND COMMUNITY VIOLENCE

	Family Conflict	
Community Violence	Severe	Minor
Victimization	.44***	.34**
Witnessing	.37**	.35**
Severe	.29*	.30*
Less severe	.36**	.34**
Moderate	.31*	.37**
Hearing about	.20	.22
Severe	.16	.24
Less severe	.16	.30*
Moderate	.16	.23

*p < .05, **p < .01, ***p < .005, (based on two-tailed tests).

be seen in Table 4, especially for victimization and witnessing, there were significant relationships between both severe and minor family conflict and community violence. Although it was not possible to separate community from family violence on the Survey of Community Violence, because of the way the questions were asked, the highly significant relationships found between these variables would suggest that it would be an important area to pursue more carefully in future studies.

In examining the Child Behavior Checklist (CBCL), 45% of the scores of the children in this sample fell at or within the clinical range for behavior problems on this measure. While few significant relationships were found between the Survey

Table 5

CORRELATIONS BETWEEN CBCL, COMMUNITY VIOLENCE
AND FAMILY CONFLICT

	CBCL		
	Total	Internal	External
Community Violence			
Victimization	.25	.25	.24
Severe	.09	.11	.24
Less severe	.22	.20	.22
Moderate	.29*	.33*	.24
Witnessing	.25	.30*	.20
Severe	.07	.14	.02
Less severe	.26	.26	.24
Moderate	.19	.21	.14
Hearing about	.16	.15	.15
Severe	.12	.10	.10
Less severe	.07	.04	.07
Moderate	.07	.08	.04
Family Conflict			
Severe	.67***	.68***	.64***
Minor	.37**	.34*	.41***
Age Parenting Began	−.31*	−.24	−.32*

*p < .05, **p < .01, ***p < .005, (based on two-tailed tests).

of Exposure to Community Violence and the CBCL for either Total or Internalizing and Externalizing scores, strong relationships were found between reported minor and severe family conflicts on the Conflict Tactics Scale and behavior problems in the children on the CBCL (see Table 5).

CBCL scores were also significantly related to the age at which parenting began, with higher behavior problem scores being associated with children of younger mothers for the total score ($r = -.31$) and the externalizing score ($r = -.32$). Again, the effectiveness of using multiple variables in predicting CBCL total scores was examined with a stepwise multiple regression procedure. Results of the stepwise analysis indicated that two variables, severe family conflict ($r = .70$) and age at which parenting began ($r = -.39$), accounted for 54% of the variance in CBCL scores ($R = .73$, $F = 26.08$, $p < .001$). Separate analyses with CBCL internalizing and externalizing scores showed similar findings.

DISCUSSION

The results of this survey of exposure to community violence for elementary school children living in a high-violence area indicated that these youngsters not only heard about a great deal of violence but witnessed much severe violence and were frequently victims of less severe forms of violence. The results also showed strong and significant relationships between reports of intrafamily violence and exposure to community violence. Based on the way the Survey of Community Violence was written and analyzed, it was not possible to differentiate clearly whether the violence was perpetrated by a family member or non-family member. This is an issue that should be investigated more carefully in future studies in order to differentiate the effects on the children of personal versus indirect exposure to family violence. The findings from the present study point to the potential importance of this association in relation to both reports of stress symptoms and child behavior problems.

Strong evidence was found in the present study indicating that stress reactions in the children are related to violence exposure. While significant relationships were not found between violence exposure and behavior problems reported in the children, they were found between indices of family conflict and reported behavior problems. Because almost half of this sample fell at or within the clinical range on the CBCL, the more limited variability of the scores may have contributed to the lack of relationship between exposure to violence and reported behavior problems. Alternatively, the impact of community violence on child behavior might be mediated by the family since family conflict resolution was related to both violence exposure and child behavior. The effects of community violence on the incidence of problem behaviors in children and, as mentioned earlier, the relationship between family violence exposure and community violence exposure are areas that need to be studied more intensively in future work with more specific behavioral and clinical assessments.

What do these findings mean for the children and their mental health? We are only at the preliminary stages of learning about the effects of chronic community violence on children. However, we do know – based on observations of children growing up in neighborhoods with much violence, as well as children exposed to other types of violence (i.e., sniper attacks) – that behaviors that are of concern develop after such experiences (Pynoos et al. 1987).

In addition to responding to the study measures, the mothers in our sample talked with us about their children's exposure to violence, their feelings about it, and the ways they tried to handle the problem. As they reported on their children's exposure to these various forms of violence, there was often a matter-of-fact quality to their reports as they reiterated numerous examples of violence, likely related to living with so much violence. The mothers reported teaching their children to sit in their homes or watch television with their heads below the window sills in order to avoid random bullets. Children learn to dive or run when they hear shots. Very early in their lives, children must learn to deal with loss and cope with grieving over and over for family members or friends who have been killed. One teenager, who escaped to a safer high school but still lived in the neighborhood, said to his mother sadly that most of the boys he grew up with were dead and he didn't know how to deal with his feelings. His mother also felt helpless in trying to work with him in dealing with such trauma.

Mothers reported that children who were previously happy became sad, angry, aggressive, tough, and seemingly uncaring. It is possible that children also experience conflicting and confusing feelings, with an increased need to seek comfort from their mothers but also anger because of feeling that they were not protected by their mothers in the first place. Other behaviors of concern have been reported, including disturbances of affect, sleep disturbances, nightmares, difficulties in peer relations, and erratic behaviors. Based on available studies and reports, many of which were reviewed in the introductory section of this paper, it can be concluded that the following behaviors might be expected to occur more often in children living in situations of chronic violence:

1. In school, they may have difficulty concentrating because of both lack of sleep and intrusive imagery.
2. They may also experience memory impairment because of avoidance or intrusive thoughts.
3. They may develop anxious attachment with their mothers, being fearful of leaving them or sleeping alone.
4. Their play may become more aggressive related to imitating behaviors they have seen as well as showing a desperate effort to protect themselves.
5. They may "act tough" to deal with their fear, developing a counterphobic reaction.
6. They may act uncaring because of having to deal with so much hurt and loss.

7. They may become severely constricted in activities, exploration, and thinking for fear of reexperiencing the traumatic event.

Perhaps worthy of note, based on our studies of adolescent mothers (Osofsky et al. in press) and those of others, we know that almost half of the children at risk for exposure to community violence in many communities have been parented by adolescent mothers. In addition to exposure to community violence, based on informal reports from child abuse and mental health clinics, the children of adolescent mothers are frequently seen as victims of child abuse and are seen in mental health clinics with significant behavioral and personality problems. Our current CBCL findings indicate that these already more vulnerable children, who are then exposed to chronic community violence, may develop additional stress-related symptoms. It is likely that their symptoms and probable behavioral problems would benefit from appropriate interventions. In addition to focusing on children who are exposed to chronic violence in general, it may be important to target groups with underlying vulnerability, such as children of adolescent mothers who are then exposed to chronic community violence.

In conclusion, through our survey of the effects of community violence on a group of elementary school children in New Orleans, we have gained information about a relatively unexplored area of significant importance for the mental health of children growing up in our country today. In most of our major cities across the country, a high proportion of our poor children are living in such environments. We must not only raise awareness about the magnitude and urgency of the problem, but continue with more intensive research to refine our understanding of the outcomes of such exposure and facilitate intervention efforts. We must learn more about what can be done to prevent increasingly difficult adjustment and problems for these children in the future.

REFERENCES

ACHENBACH, T. M., and EDELBROCK, C. S. Behavioral problems and competencies reported by parents of normal and disturbed children aged four through sixteen. *Monographs of the Society for Research in Child Development* (1981) 46:Serial No. 188.

FREDERICK, C. Children traumatized by catastrophic situations. In J. Laube and S. A. Murphy, eds., *Perspectives on Disaster Recovery* (pp. 110-30). Appleton-Century-Crofts, 1985.

KRAMER, M., SCHOEN, L. S., and KINNEY, L. The dream experience in dream-disturbed Vietnam veterans. In B. Van der Kolk, ed., *Post-Traumatic Stress Disorder: Psychological and Biological Sequelae* (pp. 82-95). American Psychiatric Press, 1984.

KRISTAL, L. Bruxism: An anxiety response to environmental stress. In C. Spielberger, I. Sarason, and F. Milgram, eds., *Stress and Anxiety*, Vol. 8. Hemisphere, 1982.

MARTINEZ, P., and RICHTERS, J. E. The NIMH community violence project: II. Children's distress symptoms associated with violence exposure. *Psychiatry* (1993) 56:22-35.

OSOFSKY, J. D., HANN, D. M., and PEEBLES, C. Adolescent parenthood: Risks and opportunities for mothers and their infants. In C. Zeanah, ed., *Handbook of Infant Mental Health*. Guilford Publications, in press.

PYNOOS, R. S., and NADER, K. Case study: Children's memory and proximity to violence. *American Academy of Child and Adolescent Psychiatry* (1989) 28:236-41.

PYNOOS, R., NADER, K., FREDERICK, C., GONDA, L., and STUBER, M. Grief reactions in school age children following a sniper attack at school. *Israeli Journal of Psychiatry & Related Sciences* (1987) 24:53-63.

RICHTERS, J. E. *Children's Stress Symptoms—Parent Report*. Unpublished measure, Child and Adolescent Disorders Research Branch, NIMH, 1990.

RICHTERS, J. E, and MARTINEZ, P. The NIMH community violence project: I. Children as victims of and witnesses to violence. *Psychiatry* (1993) 56: 7-21.

RICHTERS, J. E., and SALTZMAN, W. *Survey of Exposure to Community Violence—Parent Report Version*. Unpublished measure, Child and Adolescent Disorders Research, NIMH, 1990.

STRAUS, M. A. Measuring intrafamily conflict and violence: The Conflict Tactics Scale. *Journal of Marriage and the Family* (1979) 41:75-88.

TERR, L. *Too Scared to Cry*. Harper & Row, 1990.

Community Violence and Children on Chicago's Southside

Carl C. Bell and Esther J. Jenkins

THIS report summarizes a program of study on African-American children and violence conducted by a comprehensive community mental health center on the southside of Chicago. The research, which looked at exposure to violence, self-reports of aggression, and possible interventions, grew out of: (1) an awareness of the enormous amount of familial and extrafamilial violence in the black community; (2) clinical experiences that indicated that victimization and covictimization (i.e., victimization of close others) were often significant factors in the lives of the mentally ill; (3) a growing uneasiness, and indeed curiosity, over the extent to which children were witnessing these events and the impact of this witnessing, particularly on their own levels of aggression; and (4) a belief that the integrity of the black community was being threatened by the violence and that solutions must be sought.

Violence is a major problem in African-American communities, particularly in the inner city. Homicide rates for African-Americans are six to seven times greater than that for whites (Fingerhut and Kleinman 1990; Griffith and Bell 1989). In fact, homicide is the leading cause of death for black males and females between the ages of 15 and 34 (Griffith and Bell 1989). Furthermore, the amount of near lethal violence is many times that of the homicide rate. Estimates of the assault-to-homicide ratio are as high as 100 to 1 (Rosenberg and Mercy 1986). A comparison of lethal and potentially lethal violence in Chicago in 1990 shows that for every homicide that occurred there were 44 instances of assault serious enough to warrant police intervention (Recktenwald 1991).

Violence and mayhem is not evenly distributed across all neighborhoods and demographic groups. Evidence suggests that it occurs in inner-city neighborhoods, disproportionately among the young and in public places. In Chicago in 1990, the homicide rate ranged from 106 per 100,000 in the most violent police district to 2.1 murders in the least violent district (Chicago Police Department 1990). The six areas with the highest crime rates were also the poorest areas in the city (Recktenwald 1991). In other cities similar patterns occur where relatively small areas of the city contribute disproportionately to the violent crime rate ("A Tour of the Urban Killing Fields" 1989).

Much of the record increase is accounted for by homicide among males 20 years of age and younger (Centers for Disease Control 1990). In Chicago, approxi-

Carl C. Bell, MD, is Associate Professor of Clinical Psychiatry, University of Illinois School of Medicine, Chicago; Executive Director, Community Mental Health Council, Inc., Chicago, Illinois.

Esther J. Jenkins, PhD, is Professor of Psychology, Chicago State University, Chicago; Research Director, Community Mental Health Council, Inc., Chicago, Illinois.

mately 30% of last year's homicides involved victims age 20 and younger, and 44% of the perpetrators were age 20 and younger (Chicago Police Department 1990). Looking at firearm deaths alone, these percentages represent a 58% increase in victims in this age group over the previous year and a 48% increase in perpetrators. Most distressingly, since our first survey in 1985 there has been a 265% increase in firearm deaths of 0- to 20-year-olds (79 to 209) and a 324% increase in perpetrators (100 to 324) with most of that increase occurring since 1989 (Chicago Police Department 1990).

Furthermore, the violence that occurs is distressingly public. An analysis of 1990 Chicago murders by location shows that 538 of the 851 total were committed outdoors, with 432 occurring in a "public way" (i.e., street, alley, park). An additional 35 occurred in public housing buildings and 214 occurred in a residence (Chicago Police Department 1990).

A picture emerges from the homicide/violence statistics of neighborhoods with rampant violence occurring in situations that, at the least, can be observed by a number of people, and at worst, that endanger bystanders. Against this backdrop, it is not surprising that Dubrow and Garbarino (1989), in an informal sample of 10 mothers in a Chicago public housing development, found that all of the children had a first-hand encounter with a shooting by age 5.

EXPOSURE-TO-VIOLENCE STUDIES

Our research on children primarily has examined prevalence of exposure to violence — as a witness, victim, or having knowledge of close others' victimization — in elementary and high school children, psychiatric outpatients, and medical outpatients. In addition, we have explored perpetration and correlates of self-reported aggression in elementary school children, and have evaluated a violence intervention for these children and their parents. With the exception of the work with the elementary school children, the data collections have been adjunct to services for the children (i.e., workshop, medical treatment, therapy). All of the data collections were intended to provide information that could be used in designing or refining clinical programs. The number of children in the four samples — (total N = 1762) witnessing, knowing of others being victimized, personally being victimized, and victimizing others — are presented in Table 1.

Survey of Elementary School Children

Our first survey on children and violence was an exploratory survey of 536 elementary school children that examined children's witnessing of violence, their own involvement in arguments and fights, and a number of demographic and background variables (Jenkins and Thompson 1986; Jenkins, Thompson, and Mokros, unpublished). The children were second (n = 150), fourth (n = 100), sixth (n = 143), and eighth (n = 143) graders at three inner-city grade schools. The sample was 54% male. While children were not asked about family income, an analysis of census data indicated that the schools were located within areas with median incomes ranging from marginally above that of the entire city to 23% below that of the city (but none below the poverty level for a family of four). In addition, the schools were located in police districts with moderate (at the median) levels of homicide.

A 32-item questionnaire, developed for use in this study, was administered in small-group settings. The children were asked if they had witnessed fighting and arguing between parents, other relatives and friends; if they had seen someone shot, stabbed, beaten, or robbed in real life; and the frequency with which they engaged in fights and arguments. In addition to demographics, the children were asked about other variables related to aggression: father's presence, physical pun-

Table 1

KNOWLEDGE OF WITNESSING, VICTIMIZATION, AND PERPETRATION OF VIOLENCE IN FOUR SAMPLES
OF AFRICAN-AMERICAN ADOLESCENTS

	Survey[a]: 7- to 15-year-olds (N = 536)		Screening[b]: 10- to 19-year-olds (N = 997)		Psychiatric Outpatients[c] <18 years old (N = 84)		Medical Outpatients[c] <18 years old (N = 83)	
	n	(%)	n	(%)	n	(%)	n	(%)
Knows someone who was:								
Robbed	—		507	(50.9)	14	(17.0)	28	(34.0)
Raped	—		134	(13.4)	19	(23.0)	10	(12.0)
Assaulted	—		—		22	(26.0)	33	(40.0)
Stabbed	—		262	(26.3)	—		—	
Shot	—		289	(29.0)	—		—	
Killed	—		—		12	(14.0)	16	(19.0)
Witnessed a:	(n = 500)		(n = 1011)					
Beating	391	(78.4)	—		—		—	
Robbery	—		557	(55.1)	—		—	
Stabbing	150	(30.0)	348	(34.6)	—		—	
Shooting	131	(26.3)	400	(39.4)	—		—	
Killing	—		236	(23.5)	—		—	
Victim of:							(n = 107)	
Robbery	—		159	(15.9)	16	(19.0)	9	(8.0)
Sexual assault	—		25	(2.5)	5	(6.0)	2	(2.0)
Physical assault	—		—		31	(37.0)	19	(18.0)
Stabbing	—		43	(4.3)	—		—	
Shooting	—		32	(3.2)	—		—	
Threatened w/knife	—		226	(22.7)	—		—	
Threatened w/gun	—		169	(17.0)	—		—	
Shot at	—		109	(10.9)	—		—	
Perpetrated:								
Knife pulling	—		154	(15.7)	—		—	
Gun pulling	—		0		—		—	
Robbery	—		35	(3.6)	—		—	
Rape	—		35	(3.6)	—		—	
Stabbing	—		88	(8.9)	—		—	
Shooting	—		—		—		—	
Frequent fights[d]	114	(21.2)	—		—		—	

[a]Jenkins and Thompson, (1986).
[b]Uehara, Chalmers, Jenkins, and Shakoor (in press).
[c]Bell, Hildreth, Jenkins, Levi, and Carter (1988).
[d]*Frequent:* once or twice a week or more.

ishment, and head trauma (being knocked unconscious).

The most surprising finding of the story was the extent to which these children had witnessed life-threatening violence. As shown in Table 1, one in four (26%) of the children reported that they had seen someone shot, and 30% reported witnessing a stabbing. Girls were as likely as boys to report having seen a stabbing or shooting; with the exception of seeing a beating, violence exposure (shootings and stabbings) was not linearly related to age for these 7- to 15-year-olds.

An analysis of the correlates of these students' self-reports of involvement in fights found that witnessing of a shooting or a stabbing was associated with more fighting, as were reports of parents' and relatives' fighting. Boys reported more frequent involvement in fights than did girls, as did younger children, children who reported being physically punished, and those from father-absent homes.

Screening of High School and Elementary School Students

As part of violence awareness and prevention workshops for public school students conducted by the Community Mental Health Council's Victims Services Program, data were collected on the participants' level of violence exposure, victimization, and perpetration (Shakoor and Chalmers 1991; Uehara, Chalmers, Jenkins, and Shakoor in press). The students were asked whether they had ever seen a robbery, shooting, stabbing, or killing and the identity of the victim; whether they had experienced any of eight types of victimization ranging from attempted rape and being threatened with a weapon to being shot or stabbed; and whether they had perpetrated any of those acts. A total of 1035 students from four high schools and two middle schools were screened. The students were from health education and social science classes, all of whom were participating in violence prevention workshops. (The data collection occurred at the beginning of the workshop.) The stu-

dents—whose ages ranged from 10 to 19 years, with a median age of 15—resided in low-income, moderate to extremely high crime areas.

Among these students, three out of four had witnessed a robbery, stabbing, shooting, and/or killing: 35% had witnessed a stabbing, 39% a shooting, and 24% reported that they had seen someone killed (see Table 1). Forty-five percent had seen more than one violent incident. Many of the victims of the observed violence were known to these children: 50% of the shooting victims were either a classmate, friend, neighbor, or family member, as were 55% of the stabbing victims and 40% of those murdered.

As shown in Table 1, almost half (47%) of these students had been personally victimized (including threatened with a weapon), with 11% reporting that they had been shot at, 3% having been shot, and 4% having been stabbed. In addition, one third (33%) of the students reported that they carried a weapon, usually a knife, with 12% indicating that they had injured someone with a knife or gun. These students' victimization and perpetration experiences were parallel: The most frequent types of victimization was being threatened with a gun (17%) or knife (23%), and the most frequently reported victimization of others was pulling a knife (16%), although none of these students reported ever having pulled a gun on anyone.

An examination of factors related to exposure found that the strongest predictor of witnessing, victimization, and perpetration was carrying a weapon. Gender and age were not related to witnessing but were related to victimization and perpetration, with older youths and males reporting more of the latter.

The students' experiences with violence were cumulative; those witnessing a killing had also witnessed less severe violence (robbery, shooting, stabbing) and those who had perpetrated a violent act also had witnessed violence and been victimized. That is, rarely did students report perpetration who had not also witnessed violence and been victimized; rarely did they report having witnessed a killing without having seen lesser types of violence. This pattern suggests immersion in a violent milieu in which children are exposed to violence and are at high risk for victimization and perpetration of violence.

Screening of Psychiatric and Medical Outpatients

Since 1984 the agency has taken a victimization history on its patients as part of the intake process. In addition to asking about personal victimizations of physical and sexual assault, the brief screening form also asks about knowledge of victimization of close others, that is, friends, family members, neighbors (Bell, Taylor-Crawford, Jenkins, and Chalmers 1988). Subsequently, the screening form was administered at an outpatient medical clinic in a high-crime, high-poverty area on the near northside of Chicago (Bell, Hildreth, Jenkins, Levi, and Carter 1988).

An analysis of data on patients 18 years of age and younger (who comprised 20% of the psychiatric group and 41% of the medical sample) found a considerable amount of personal victimization and knowledge of victimization (see Table 1). Consistent with the findings from the adult samples, the mentally ill youngsters ($n = 84$) reported more sexual and physical assault than those from the medical clinic ($n = 107$).

While these statistics reflect the greater vulnerability of the mentally ill (or possibly the role of victimization in the onset of mental illness), the data on victimization of close others are more mixed, possibly reflecting the somewhat higher crime rate of the area surrounding the medical clinic. As seen in Table 1, 23% of the mentally ill youths and 12% of the medical clinic youths knew of someone who had been raped and 19% of the medical patients and 14% of the psychiatric outpatients knew of someone who had been murdered. Interestingly, boys in both the psychiatric and medical groups were equally likely to report that a "close other" had been mur-

dered, and this percentage (9%) was considerably lower than that for girls (26% for medical clinic patients and 23% of psychiatric clinic patients).

In summary, the picture that emerges from these surveys of children and adolescents on the southside of Chicago is one of considerable exposure to violence, particularly as witnesses and "survivors" (having close others victimized). Witnessing of a shooting ranged from one in four of the second–eighth graders to approximately four in ten of the fourth through 12th graders. Almost 25% of the latter had seen someone killed. Witnessing of robberies was quite common, although we do not know if these robberies involved use of force. Almost 30% of those seen killed were family members or friends. Approximately ¼ of these kids reported that a close other was shot or stabbed, whether or not they personally witnessed the incident.

In comparison to the "normal" youth from the public school as well as the medical clinic, psychiatrically impaired youngsters and those that they knew seemed to have been at particular risk for sexual and physical assault. This finding of greater victimization of the mentally ill is consistent with research on adults (Carmen, Rieker, and Mills 1984).

In addition to generating data on the prevalence of violence exposure, each of these studies provided information about the dynamics of such encounters. Some of this information is not new: that involvement in fights is associated with younger ages (Moore and Mukai 1983), being male (Maccoby and Jacklin 1974), and the presence of physical punishment (Eron, Walder, and Lefkowitz 1971). However, the finding that children from father-absent homes were more aggressive needs follow-up study, although there is some literature that supports this result (Montare and Boone 1980). The finding that children's self-reports of fights were related to parent and other kin fighting but not to peer fighting reinforces the importance of family socialization in the development of aggressive behavior.

One of the more interesting findings of

the screening of the mentally ill youngsters and those from the medical clinic is the gender differences in awareness of others' victimization. Boys and girls were equally likely to report that they had been assaulted, but girls were more likely to know of the victimization of close others. Girls were more likely to know of others having been victimized in all of the five categories (molested, raped, robbed, assaulted, murdered) and were 2.5 to 3 times more likely to report that a close other had been murdered, with percentages comparable to that of the adult samples. While we can not rule out the explanation that these young males, for some reason, are less likely to know about others' victimizations, the findings, nonetheless, raise questions about young black males' perceptions and recall of threatening events. (An alternative explanation is that, perhaps, these young males do not equate "murdered"–which suggests an unjustified act–with "killed," which implies no such judgment about the cause of death.)

Also of considerable interest is the absence of a linear relationship between age and prevalence of witnessing violence. In the high school screening, which included students aged 10 to 19, with a median age of 15, the percentage of kids witnessing a killing ranged from 22% to 30%, in a nonlinear fashion. (Age was significantly associated with perpetration and victimization.) Among the 7- to 15-year-olds in the violence survey, age was not related to witnessing of a shooting nor of a stabbing. The suggestion is that shootings are so prevalent in these communities that initial exposure occurs at an early age. (One would, however, expect to find a relationship between frequency of exposure and age.)

Finally, the finding that witnessing, victimization, and perpetration are cumulative helps to clarify the victimization–perpetration relationship. It is consistent with previous findings on the overlap between victims and offenders in adult populations (Dennis et al. 1981; Rose 1981) and suggests strategies for intervention. If histories of victimization are, in many instances, precursors to perpetration,

then victims should be treated as "at risk" for committing future violence.

The findings from these studies are consistent with others in the field and, we believe, provide useful information in this understudied but critical area. However, the studies have many of the methodological flaws noted by Widom (1989) that typically characterize cycle-of-violence studies. The limitations of these studies include the reliance on self-report, retrospective data that may be subject to recall errors, and the absence of appropriate comparison groups. (However, it is not clear how one would go about getting a reliable corroboration of exposure to street violence, particularly for adolescents.) Individual students' interpretations of events, particularly "robbed," may vary. In addition, the studies were done with convenience samples rather than randomly selected ones. Thus, the results must be interpreted with caution and, in the final analysis, are most useful in providing directions for future research under more controlled circumstances.

INTERVENTION RETREAT

In addition to studies on exposure, the agency implemented and evaluated a workshop designed to explore nonviolent approaches to conflict resolution. A total of 40 children and 35 adults attended the workshop, about half of whom were volunteers from the "Survey of Elementary Schools" described previously. While small in scope (although quite ambitious from other perspectives), the intervention yielded useful information about intervention strategies.

The intervention consisted of a day-and-a-half retreat for the families (all children had to be accompanied by an adult) at which dramatizations of violent and potentially violent situations were presented to the entire group. The skits were followed by small-group discussions on the implications of the dramatized events and constructive ways of handling the situation. All participants completed a preretreat questionnaire and a postretreat questionnaire, and 90% were interviewed by phone a year after the retreat. (The retreat was conducted in summer 1985.)

Overall, the results of the evaluation indicated that the retreat per se was not that effective in altering attitudes about violent solutions to conflict. For example, 89% of the adults indicated they would talk to an attacker, up from 75% in the preretreat questionnaire. However, a year later only 62% of these respondents were willing to talk in response to an attack. Willingness to fight followed a similar pattern, as did willingness to get a weapon to protect oneself.

A different pattern of responses emerged for the children. While there was no difference in children's reported inclinations to talk vs. fight if attacked, from preretreat to immediate postretreat, responses had moved toward a more nonviolent posture 1 year later. This "delayed reaction" suggests that the changes were a result of maturation rather than treatment.

While the retreat did not produce immediate and dramatic results, explanations of its evaluation's findings suggest useful information about interventions that were subsequently incorporated into our intervention efforts. For example, there were greater changes in attitudes and behaviors that were most clearly and specifically addressed at the retreat. At postretreat, participants were less likely to indicate they would use a weapon in response to threat and more likely to indicate they would call police in response to a fight – both frequent themes of the sessions. That the participants often had very different reactions to the information (some moving from violent to nonviolent responses while others actually did the reverse), raises the question whether the impact of the information was mediated by personality variables and/or personal circumstances. That is, individuals who have been victimized, have a history of perpetration, or have a tendency toward fear and anxiety may respond very differently to "consciousness raising" information on

the incidence and prevalence of interpersonal violence in their communities.

The agency is concerned about raising the awareness of those who work with children regarding the pernicious effects of violence exposure and also to encourage others, particularly those providing direct service, to do research in this area. One such effort resulted in some interesting and useful case studies by a school social worker (Dyson 1990), who noted that all six of the young African-American boys individually referred to her for their behavioral problems had experienced the murder of at least one close family member. Furthermore, the children's grieving process had been complicated by accompanying rage over the manner in which their kin had died. Using a posttraumatic stress disorder (PTSD) paradigm, the youths' issues were addressed in group and individual sessions, and considerable improvement was accomplished.

Research efforts such as this one provide enormously useful data and insightful interpretations, while sharpening the practitioners' conceptualization of the problem/issues. However, although many practitioners are quite capable of doing quality research, more often than not the process is greatly facilitated by collaborations with academicians, who typically have greater resources and expertise in the research area.

CONCLUSIONS

Clearly, research in the area of children and community violence is just beginning as we move beyond basic questions of prevalence of exposure to more complicated ones of buffers, mediating factors, and consequences. For example, the work of Pynoos and others (Pynoos and Eth 1985; Pynoos and Nader 1990; Terr 1991) indicates that a frequent response to violence exposure is posttraumatic stress disorder symptoms, the manifestation of which varies by developmental level, physical closeness to the incident, and emotional closeness to victim. How are these symptoms affected by the repeated exposure to violence that often characterizes the lives of inner-city children? How is the experience of violence exposure and coping affected by poverty and its attendant negative life events that these children and their families experience? Are there personality and/or familial characteristics that either shield children from exposure to chronic violence in dangerous neighborhoods and/or that help them cope effectively with the experience once it occurs? What happens to children who experience both chronic community violence and familial violence?

The issue of poor, young black males' functioning in a violent milieu is of particular concern. With the highest rates of school drop-out and unemployment (Wilson 1987) and the most rapidly increasing rates of victimization and perpetration (Centers for Disease Control 1990; Chicago Police Department 1990), the very survival of this group is threatened. Although girls and boys do not seem to differ greatly in witnessing lethal violence, statistics on victim characteristics indicate that the victims witnessed are most likely young males. How does this very real threat, often underscored by frequent attendance at peers' funerals, affect adolescent males' sense of a future? How does a sense of future impact on willingness to engage in risk-taking behaviors, including violence? How is a willingness to form close relationships with others affected when you are not sure about your own future or that of the other person? Questions of future orientation and object relations (see Terr 1991) are particularly relevant for poor, young black males, who may already feel alienated from a society that is not making a place for them and for whom the adolescent tendency toward risk taking can be exacerbated by attempts to compensate for societal barriers to achievement. When does a sense of futurelessness turn into nihilism? Which violence interventions strategies work best for these groups?

Are there gender differences in the impact of witnessing violence and of living in a violent milieu in which young black males die disproportionately? Does such exposure also impact on adolescent females' sense of future and object relations as they experience the loss of mates and potential mates?

Answers to these and the many unasked questions about impact of exposure are important to developing interventions, primary and secondary, for children who live in these high-risk environments. It is essential that we recognize and treat the deleterious effects of violence exposure. It is even more critical, however, that we dramatically reduce the amount of violence in inner-city communities that is threatening a generation of black youth as victims, covictims, and perpetrators.

REFERENCES

BELL, C. C., HILDRETH, C. J., JENKINS, E. J., LEVI, D., and CARTER, C. The need for victimization screening in a poor, outpatient medical population. *Journal of the National Medical Association* (1988) 80:853-60.

BELL, C. C., TAYLOR-CRAWFORD, K., JENKINS, E. J., and CHALMERS, D. Need for victimization screening in a black psychiatric population. *Journal of the National Medical Association* (1988) 80: 41-48.

CARMEN, E., RIEKER, P. P., and MILLS, T. Victims of violence and psychiatric illness. *American Journal of Psychiatry* (1984) 141:378-83.

CENTER FOR DISEASE CONTROL. Homicide among young Black Males — United States, 1978-1987.

Morbidity and Mortality Weekly Report (1990) 39: 869-73.

CHICAGO POLICE DEPARTMENT. *Murder Analysis.* Detective Division, Chicago Police Department, 1990.

DENNIS, R. E., KIRK, A., and KNUCKLES, B. N. *Black Males at Risk to Low Life Expectancy: A Study of Homicide Victims and Perpetrators.* National Institute of Mental Health, Center for Studies of Minority Group Mental Health, 1981.

DUBROW, N. F., and GARBARINO, J. Living in the war zone: Mothers and young children in public housing development. *Journal of Child Welfare* (1989) 68:3-20.

DYSON, J. L. The effect of family violence on children's academic performance and behavior. *Journal of the National Medical Association* (1990) 82: 17–22.

ERON, L., WALDER, L. O., and LEFKOWITZ, M. *Learning of Aggression in Childhood*. Little, Brown, 1971.

FINGERHUT, L. A., and KLEINMAN, J. C. International and interstate comparisons of homicide among young males. *Journal of the American Medical Association* (1990) 263:3292–95.

GRIFFITH, E. H., and BELL, C. C. Recent trends in suicide and homicide among Blacks. *Journal of the American Medical Association* (1989) 262:2265–69.

JENKINS, E. J., and THOMPSON, B. *Children talk about violence: Preliminary findings from a survey of black elementary school children*. Presented at the Nineteenth Annual Convention of the Association of Black Psychologists, Oakland, CA, 1986.

JENKINS, E. J., THOMPSON, B., and MOKROS, H. *Correlates of self-perceived aggression black children*. Unpublished.

MACCOBY, E. E., and JACKLIN, C. N. *The Psychology of Sex Differences*. Stanford University Press, 1974.

MONTARE, A., and BOONE, S. Aggression and paternal absence: Racial ethnic differences among inner-city boys. *Journal of Genetic Psychology* (1980) 137:223–32.

MOORE, D., and MUKAI, L. Aggressive behavior in the home as a function on the age and sex of control, problem and normal children. *Journal of Abnormal Child Psychology* (1983) 11:257–72.

PYNOOS, R., and ETH, S. Developmental perspectives on psychic trauma in childhood. In R. Figley, ed., *Trauma and Its Wake*. Brunner/Mazel, 1985.

PYNOOS, R. S., and NADER, K. Children's exposure to violence and traumatic death. *Psychiatric Annals* (1990) 20:334–44.

RECKTENWALD, W. City's top crime rates still haunt poor areas. *The Chicago Tribune* (1991, April 15) Sec. 1, p. 1; Sec. 2, p. 5.

ROSE, H. M. *Black Homicide in the Urban Environment*. National Institute of Mental Health, Center for Studies of Minority Group Mental Health, 1981.

ROSENBERG, M. L., and MERCY, J. A. Homicide: Epidemiologic analysis at the national level. *Bulletin of the New York Academy of Medicine* (1986) 62: 376–99.

SHAKOOR, B. H., and CHALMERS, D. Covictimization of African-American children who witness violence and the theoretical implications of its effects on their cognitive, emotional, and behavioral development. *Journal of the National Medical Association* (1991) 83:233–38.

TERR, L. Childhood traumas: An outline and overview. *American Journal of Psychiatry* (1991) 148: 10–20.

Tour of urban killing fields. *Newsweek* (1989, January 16) p. 45.

UEHARA, E., CHALMERS, D., JENKINS, E. J., and SHAKOOR, B. Youth encounters with violence: Results from the Chicago Community Mental Health Council Violence Screening Project. *Journal of Black Studies* in press.

WIDOM, C. S. Does violence beget violence? A critical examination of the literature. *Psychological Bulletin* (1989) 109:3–28.

WILSON, W. *The Truly Disadvantaged*. University of Chicago Press, 1987.

Children's Exposure to Community Violence: Following a Path from Concern to Research to Action

Raymond P. Lorion and William Saltzman

THIS paper discusses the antecedents and current progress of an ongoing program of research on the nature, extent, and consequences of children's direct and indirect exposure to violent events and settings. Involvement in such research has sensitized the authors to difficult ethical and methodological challenges that, we believe, merit consideration by mental health scientists and policy makers. Resolution of those challenges has substantive implications for both subsequent research and the application of resultant findings.

VIOLENCE AS A MULTILEVEL PHENOMENON

The focus of this work, urban violence, is itself not a recent phenomenon (Dennis, Kirk, and Knuckles 1981; Gibbs 1984; Wilson 1975). What is new, however, is the sudden acceleration of its scope and severity in major urban areas across the nation. Increasingly, violence is experienced in some settings as nearly continuous series of random and threatening events. Anecdotal reports suggest that residents experience the atmosphere within such settings with a pervasive sense of fear, vulnerability, and hopelessness. Repeatedly, existence within such neighborhoods has been described as "living in a battle zone" and "surviving in a free-fire zone."

If such reports are valid, mental health researchers must devise strategies for confirming the existence and emotional and behavioral implications of what are likely to be significant added risk factors confronting disadvantaged families. To-ward that end, work presented herein summarizes preliminary efforts to move from anecdote to systematic estimates of the prevalence of encounters with violence in the lives of a selected sample of preadolescent urban children. Findings obtained thus far confirm both the pervasiveness of violence in the lives of these children and the emotional costs of such encounters. Unquestionably, our measurement strategies require further refinement. Nevertheless, we have confidence that those refinements will confirm the validity of our observations to this point.

As we proceed, we expect that obtained prevalence estimates and related ethnographic information can be combined to organize a taxonomy of violent encounters. In turn, the elements of that taxonomy need to be linked with their immediate and long-term emotional and behavioral consequences. It is evident already that we need to assess the impacts of violence at the community, the familial, and the individual levels.

Raymond P. Lorion, PhD, is with the Department of Psychology, University of Maryland.
William Saltzman is with the University of Maryland.
Send requests for reprints to: Raymond P. Lorion, PhD, Department of Psychology, University of Maryland, College Park, MD 20742.

We sense, for example, that pervasive violence contaminates the community within which it occurs. Thus, research must determine the ecological characteristics of such toxic environments. A potential result may be the creation of behavior settings (Barker 1978) that draw forth pathogenic individual (and, perhaps, familial) response patterns ranging from vigilance, interpersonal withdrawal, suspicion, and resignation to reduced impulse control, increased risk taking, and retaliatory or even anticipatory violence. If such behavior settings do exist, the seeds for an expansive and self-perpetuating environment of violence lie within contemporary urban settings. Interventions must be designed that simultaneously interrupt the emergence of that potential and, relatedly, ameliorate existing consequences for individuals of pervasive community violence.

At the family level, we assume that such encounters have systemic effects on family processes and relationship patterns. Maslow's (1970) hierarchy of needs may be quite salient to understanding the lives of such parents. Already strained by economic disadvantage, a family's nurturing and protective capacities may be further disrupted or incapacitated by existence within an environment of violence in which issues of safety and survival take precedence. The ability to nurture, protect, and reassure a child may be stretched for a parent who is equally at physical risk and thereby emotionally drained. Parental efficacy and authority may, in turn, be further diluted when children recognize a parent's inability to provide security and reassurance.

Thus, the conditions that force parents to choose between providing security and supervision or food and shelter for one's child(ren) may result in the need for comprehensive interventions targeted to entire families. In cases where existing family resources are adequate to protect the child(ren), interventions may be needed to relieve the emotional strain on the parent(s) of providing such protection. It needs to be recognized that some families

cope effectively and independently with such stressful environments. Understanding how they do so can enhance the ecological validity (Bronfenbrenner 1977; Lorion 1990) of potential interventions.

At the individual level, research on the emotional and behavioral consequences of exposure to violence for individual children provides only limited insights into both its consequences and underlying mechanisms. As noted below, being reared in violent settings can significantly distort "normal" developmental sequences. Children from such environments, for example, may present the cumulative effects of a series of negatively resolved psychosocial crises (Erikson 1963). Exposure to pervasive violence may leave children with tentative senses of basic trust, autonomy, and initiative. With such an inadequate psychosocial foundation, adolescents would be challenged to overcome feelings of inferiority and role confusion, and unprepared to resolve issues of intimacy and generativity.

Ultimately, a portion of the generation raised in violent settings may confront quite early that psychosocial crisis described by Erikson (1963) as "despair.' Unlike the elderly who suffer from the perception that insufficient time remains to compensate for incompletely achieved goals, children of violence may despairingly conclude that, time available notwithstanding, they have neither the resources nor the likelihood of achieving lasting or socially approved outcomes. For them, socially unacceptable and risky, albeit immediately rewarding, alternatives may become highly attractive. In turn, their choices may perpetuate that very environment of violence that limited their options.

CHILDREN'S EXPOSURE TO VIOLENCE

The mental health disciplines are presently limited in both their knowledge of and capacity to respond to this phenomenon. Crisis theory and crisis intervention techniques (Slaikeu 1990) provide, respectively, insights into and options for responding to emotional trauma resulting generally from violent *episodes*. Yet, the phenomenon of interest is chronic, environmentally pervasive violence. As such, concern must be extended beyond the direct victims of violent events to include those *indirectly affected* because they have witnessed such events or because such events have occurred to members of their immediate and extended family or acquaintances. Indirect victims, we believe, also include those who have personalized the threat of violence because of its seeming frequency, ubiquity, and unpredictability within their communities.

Some findings related to this broadened definition of childhood "victims of violence" can be found. Dubrow and Garbarino (1989) and Bell and Jenkins (1990) have noted, for example, that children are frequently present when violence occurs among adult family members or acquaintances. Pynoos and Eth (1985) have estimated that children may be witness to approximately 20% of the homicides occurring in Los Angeles County. Surveying more than 500 elementary school children living in violent neighborhoods in Chicago, Jenkins and Thompson (1986) found that nearly one in four had personally witnessed an aggravated assault.

In their sample of 1000 African-American elementary and high school students, Shakoor and Chalmers (1991) found that nearly three in four reported having witnessed at least one instance of someone being robbed, stabbed, shot, or killed. In one elementary school participating in this survey, 85% of the children stated that they had witnessed some form of violent crime. Nearly half (47%) of the students in this sample claimed to have experienced directly events ranging from being threatened with a gun or knife to being robbed, raped, or shot.

Building on their pioneering work studying the psychological status of children living in war-torn areas such as Africa, Asia, and the Middle East (Garbarino, Kostelny, and Dubrow 1989, 1991, 1992), Garbarino and his colleagues have

conducted detailed interviews of children and families living in disadvantaged sections of Chicago. In one community, for example, *all* children interviewed reported that they had witnessed a shooting before the age of 5 (Dubrow and Garbarino 1989). In such communities, it was observed that children instinctively dropped to the ground at the sound of gunfire and were trained to keep low and avoid windows when indoors.

Reflecting on their experiences across multiple settings, Garbarino, Kostelny, and Dubrow (1991) have noted similarities between the lives of children encountering urban violence and children living in combat areas. It appears that exposure to chronic danger typically necessitates developmental accommodations with pervasive effects on interpersonal, cognitive, behavioral, and psychological processes (Dubrow and Garbarino 1989). Noted effects appear to be both cumulative and enduring (Dubrow and Garbarino 1989; Pynoos et al. 1987). Included among these effects are regressive behaviors such as enuresis and thumb sucking, continuing feelings of anxiety and helplessness, and even emotional numbness. Problems with attention and concentration as well as general academic performance have also been noted (Bell and Jenkins 1990; Pynoos and Nader, 1988).

Garbarino, Kostelny, and Dubrow (1992) have also described a category of pathological adaptation to chronic violence. Included within this category are conditions involving generalized desensitization to the threat and consequences of violence, and an almost addictive pursuit of opportunities for risk taking and confrontation with danger. One might speculate that such a pattern represents a behavioral manifestation of the "despair" described earlier. Without hope for the future, some individuals may attempt to gain a sense of control over their lives through repeated encounters with life-threatening situations. It may make little sense to be careful for oneself or others if physical harm or death are deemed inevitable.

As noted, evidence of such effects has primarily been reported by investigators studying the lives of children in war zones. Work by Garbarino and his colleagues documenting such effects offers heuristically valuable insights for conceptualizing and conducting studies of children exposed to pervasive urban violence. Also relevant to this research focus is a study of 159 children enrolled in an elementary school at which a sniper shooting occurred (Pynoos et al. 1987; Nader, Pynoos, Fairbanks, and Frederick 1988).

Interviews with these children and their families identified a range of psychological consequences of such exposure including intrusive imagery, anxiety, interpersonal withdrawal, sleep disorders, and attentional deficits. The investigators also observed that factors such as a child's physical proximity to the shooting, familiarity with its victims, and exposure to other traumatic events (e.g., parental separation or a physical injury) during the year preceding the shooting related to the nature and severity of observed symptoms. Direct relationships were consistently found between the degree of a child's exposure to the violent event and the severity of consequent impairment (Pynoos and Nader 1988, 1989).

Noteworthy for the study of the psychological consequences of exposure to pervasive urban violence are the following general conclusions derived from Pynoos et al.'s work: (1) proximity to the occurrence of violence relates to its potential harmfulness; (2) familiarity with a victim of violence represents one avenue through which violence can have indirect effects; and (3) repeated exposure to traumatic events serves to increase one's vulnerability for psychological and developmental sequelae rather than to inoculate one against further harm. If confirmed in direct studies of children's exposure to enduring and pervasive urban violence, these patterns would argue strongly both for intensifying our understanding of the consequences of such exposure and, as quickly as possible, for implementing and evaluating preventive interventions.

PRELIMINARY STEPS IN OUR RESEARCH

It would be misleading to suggest that our inquiries into children's exposure to violence were planned from the outset. In collaboration with local schools, we were involved in the conduct of large-scale surveys of substance involvement among preadolescent and adolescent children. Focus group interviews conducted with fourth and fifth graders as part of our measurement development steps produced what were initially interpreted as exaggerated accounts by children of their encounters with violence. Many children reported having witnessed or experienced extremely violent or threatening incidents. Some described local shootings, assaults, and a range of violent activities occurring as part of neighborhood drug dealings. They described their fears of being shot, kidnapped, or hurt when outside in their neighborhoods.

The number of such spontaneous comments led us to examine their accuracy. Both spontaneously and in response to specific questions, teachers, principals, and other school administrators repeatedly commented on the number of their students whose lives seemed analogous to civilians trapped in a war zone. In spite of long experience in recognizing and responding to the demands of inner-city life on children, teachers seemed unprepared for the levels of children's fear, displaced anger, and desperation. With unexpected frequency, educators reported that responding to children's encounters as victims or witnesses of violence took precedence over cherished academic objectives.

Repeatedly, we heard that children living in violent settings would arrive at school in distress and unable to focus on schoolwork. School staff voiced concern about their students' exposure to violence and drug-related activities in their neighborhoods. Elementary school teachers described children so afraid to return home after school that they hid in their classrooms. Some children actually pleaded not to have to take the bus home. School counselors spoke of children who had been severely traumatized after witnessing violent incidents. Principals suggested that many children from "dangerous" neighborhoods had more difficulty concentrating and maintaining appropriate classroom behavior than their peers from other neighborhoods.

Based on the children's responses and staff comments, the Prince George's Drug Interest Survey (PGDIS), originally designed to assess children's involvement with alcohol and other drugs, was expanded by seven items to gauge the prevalence of children's exposure to "risky" neighborhoods. The additional items were worded to assess the degree to which the students felt safe or threatened, and the frequency with which they had witnessed or experienced violent or drug-related activities in their neighborhood. Each item began with the stem "Where I live . . . " followed by the content of interest (e.g., "most kids my age have seen someone get hurt because of drugs"; "most kids my age are scared about people using and selling drugs"; "it is safe for kids my age to play outside").

The entire survey was administered to *all* ($N = 2717$) children enrolled in grades 4, 5, and 6 in one of six administrative areas of a large metropolitan school system. The student population of this system is primarily minority (approximately 55% African-American and 35% White) from low- to middle-income families. Significant segments of the population reside in high-density, low-income neighborhoods marked by high levels of drug-related crime and violence.

The seven neighborhood items were coded so that higher scores reflected increased awareness of danger and aggregated to form an overall index of neighborhood quality. Using a quartile approach, neighborhoods were then classified by levels ranging from I (least dangerous) to IV (most dangerous). The children's responses to both individual items and the salience of their aggregate scores for predicting both their involvement with substances and their psychological state confirmed the original anecdotal reports (Saltzman and Lorion 1990).

Nearly one in six of the fourth, fifth, and sixth graders sampled, for example, indicated that in their neighborhoods, most children their age have seen people using and selling drugs, have seen people hurt because of drugs, and have themselves been asked to help sell drugs. A similar percentage of the overall sample described their neighborhoods as being "unsafe." Nearly one in five thought that kids their age would help sell drugs if asked to do so. When responses were examined by individual schools, the nonrandomness of encounters with violence became apparent. In some schools, little experience with violence was reported. In others, up to 60% of the students reported exposure to drug-related violence and 33% described their neighborhoods as unsafe.

When neighborhood characteristics were linked to substance involvement, we learned that children from level IV neighborhoods reported significantly higher levels of exposure to drug-related activities, greater access and availability of drugs, and higher levels of current, lifetime, and intended drug and alcohol use. In fact, children living in level IV neighborhoods reported levels of drug and alcohol use *up to 10 times* that of children living in level I neighborhoods.

Clearly, our initial glimpse into children's encounters with violence confirmed the initial focus group impression that exposure for some children was intense and impactful. Moreover, the observed link between neighborhood characteristics and substance involvement reported widely in the literature on risk factors for drug use (e.g., Hawkins, Lishner, and Catalano 1985; Lorion, Bussell, and Goldberg 1991) provided some reassurance of the potential validity of our results.

Recognizing the scientific limitations of our measurement procedures and findings, we collaborated with other researchers concerned with children's exposure to community violence on the design of procedures to estimate the prevalence of such exposure and its psychological concomitants. That collaboration resulted in the Community Experience Survey, an abbreviated form of the Survey of Children's Exposure to Community Violence (Richters and Saltzman 1990). One or the other of these measures was used in three parallel inquiries into children's encounters with violence in the Metropolitan Washington, DC, area (Saltzman 1992); Washington, DC (Richters and Martinez 1993); and New Orleans (Osofsky, Wewers, Hann, Fick, and Richters 1992). The consistency of findings across these distinct studies confirms the reality of the phenomenon of pervasive community violence.

A detailed report of our findings with the Community Experience Survey is provided by Saltzman (1992) and by Saltzman and Lorion (1990). Highlights of our findings are presented herein as background to ethical and methodological concerns that have arisen about the conduct of research on this topic. As reported in Saltzman (1992), the Community Experience Survey was administered to 170 fifth and sixth graders, ages 9 to 13, enrolled in two schools selected on the basis of response patterns provided by students to the aforementioned neighborhood characteristic items. As an initial scale development step, two schools were selected in which we had a basis for assuming that students were encountering relatively high levels of pervasive community violence.

Responses obtained confirmed that assumption. Nearly four out of five students reported having been either a victim and/or witness to episodes of severe (e.g., being shot at or attacked with a knife) or moderate (e.g., being beaten, chased, or otherwise physically threatened) violence. More than one in five reported being shot at, stabbed, or attacked with a gun or knife. Nearly one in six reported having witnessed a homicide; nearly two in five reported that a family member or close acquaintance had been murdered. More than 80% reported regularly hearing the sound of gunfire in their neighborhoods,

and more than 60% reported having seen someone carrying a gun or knife. A surprisingly large proportion (38%) of all reported encounters with severe and moderate violence were chronic in nature; that is, they occurred on a monthly or more frequent basis.

In addition to the Community Experience Survey, students also completed the Checklist of Child Distress Symptoms (Richters and Martinez 1990), a measure of children's experiences relevant to indices of posttraumatic stress syndrome, and the Child Depression Inventory (Kovaks 1985). These measures were administered as preliminary probes into potential links between exposure to pervasive community violence and emotional status. Generally, findings obtained confirmed the existence of such a link.

This relationship was especially evident for that portion of children within the upper quartile of reported exposure to and encounters with forms of violence. These children's distress levels were significantly higher than their classmates having less exposure. Moreover, the data suggest that the psychological impact of such exposure may be distinct across genders. It appears that girls experience more depressive indices than boys whereas boys, owing to their greater exposure to severe forms of violence presumably, experienced somewhat more distress than girls.

Unquestionably, these preliminary findings must be replicated using psychometrically refined versions of the measures with a considerably enlarged and heterogeneous sample. That caveat notwithstanding, our findings to date are consistent with both anecdotal reports and related findings observed with children living in war zones and high-risk neighborhoods. That the investigation of this phenomenon must continue seems evident based both on what is currently known and what one might potentially learn about a critical risk factor for the psychological adjustment, indeed physical survival, of children and adolescents.

ANECDOTAL VALIDATION

Subsequent discussions of our initial findings with community residents, students, and local educators provided some degree of "face validity" for our preliminary findings. Children, for example, vividly described their neighborhoods in terms characteristic of urban battlegrounds. They treated as nothing special having witnessed a shooting, police raid, or even a dead body. Children also reported that they were strictly forbidden from leaving their homes after school. Nearby playgrounds, basketball courts, and sidewalks were off limits because of the risk of drug encounters, the dangers of "drive-by" shootings, and cross-fires. In many cases, significant portions of the neighborhood had become "free-fire zones."

With regularity, residents described nighttimes filled with sirens, yelling, and fear. Some opened their door hesitantly each morning uncertain of what had occurred in their building the night before. Adults repeatedly emphasized to children the need to be cautious. Consistent with this admonition, we heard how pieces of cardboard were strategically placed across the lower portions of windows to block out the neighborhood's harsh realities. Reportedly, doing so allowed for movement within the home with less concern of having one's shadow mistakenly targeted for a "hit." Parents and teachers noted that the cardboard also served as a constant reminder to the children of the dangers outside.

In effect, for many of these children, it mattered little whether the weather was sunny, mild, rainy, or bitter cold. They remained indoors for self-protection. For much of the time, they lived under restrictions between protective custody and house arrest. For they and their parents, the "war on drugs' was being fought by, with, and over children. Some parents commented that the war was about access to the services of youth in the drug trade, their business as drug consumers, and their bodies as soldiers. Too frequently, the innocent bystanders were young children, playing or even sleeping.

BRANCHING RESEARCH QUESTIONS

As noted, an initial goal of our work has been and remains the conduct of a large-scale, psychometrically sound survey of preadolescent children and their parents. We intend to organize the results into a taxonomy of violent events, settings, and sequelae. We also appreciate how little of the phenomenon we will actually examine and the necessity of attending to the ripples caused by children's exposure to violence. The classmates of students living in such neighborhoods, for example, may represent yet another category of "indirect" victims.

Parents forced to refuse a child's request to play outside because of unpredictable danger may also be victims. Presumably the inability to insulate one's child(ren) from the sights, sounds, and fears of unending and unpredictable urban violence has emotional and behavioral consequences for a parent. If addicted or dependent on drugs, the parenting task must become even more demanding. One must respond to potentially competing motives: the physiological need for a substance and the emotional need to nurture and protect one's offspring.

Ignoring the reactive effects of children's exposure to pervasive violence on the parents and teachers responsible for caring for those children may, from the outset, jeopardize the success of any proposed interventions. Logically, many of these caregivers may be unable to serve as the intermediaries through which intervention effects are to occur. Who can provide care when everyone available is also a victim? That is an obstacle long recognized by those involved with crisis intervention (Slaikeu 1990).

Attention must also be given to identification of the objective and subjective characteristics of violent neighborhoods and settings. How distinct are actual and perceived environmental contributors to pervasive violence? How do individual characteristics and setting characteristics "transact" (Wicker 1979)? How can individual and situational risks be combined for maximal predictive accuracy in forecasting threats to children's development?

REFLECTIONS ON THE WORK

Before proceeding with this research, we feel a responsibility to consider the wisdom of Seymour Sarason's (1984) provocative essay entitled "If it can be studied or developed, should it be?" How will the conduct of investigations on pervasive community violence affect those already victimized by such violence? Considering these questions at this point of our research may reduce somewhat the potential for us to add to the victimization of the residents of such neighborhoods.

Somehow, a process to identify intended and potential unintended consequences for the community, the schools, the neighborhoods, the families, and the children of research must be incorporated within the design of research on this phenomenon. That process may need to include both investigators and community gatekeepers who *together* consider questions such as:

a. What reactive consequences can be expected?
b. What are the critical decision points in this line of research and *whose* decisions are they?
c. How does one obtain informed consent from a "community"?
d. How does one preserve the privacy and anonymity of a community?
e. Should information be obtained about problems without a commitment to participate in its solution?
f. Who "owns" an investigation's findings and decides if they are to be published?

These reflections were not stimulated solely by our admiration for Sarason's in-sights. In large part, they arose out of the candid comments of school colleagues who exposed this aspect of their students' lives with considerable hesitancy. These colleagues cautioned that residents of a community may be understandably reluctant to reveal to outsiders the violence within their lives. The affected communities have already been stigmatized as drug ridden, decaying, and generally unsafe. Bringing public attention to actual levels of violence may only confirm and magnify existing negative views. Consequently, rather than benefiting from the research and consequent programs, the communities may, in the long run, be further isolated and avoided.

We were urged to recognize community skepticism of the motives of "interested" social scientists. Based on prior experience and stereotypes, residents of these communities may predict that problems will be revealed, hopes raised, the status quo disrupted, and little else changed. Our community colleagues were admittedly pessimistic about the final conclusions resulting from our studies. They predicted that the scope of the problem and of its solution would be deemed beyond the limits of available expertise and resources. They anticipated that the level of its complexity would require interdisciplinary cooperation as yet rarely achieved among the helping professions and thus nothing would happen.

Since presumably multiple causes for the problem would be identified, uncertainty about where to begin may postpone action indefinitely. Although oft-repeated caveats about "blaming the victim" (Ryan 1971) may again be raised by the investigators, as one member of our community noted, "in the end, somehow we'll be responsible 'cause we let it happen."

BALANCING SCIENCE AND SOCIAL NEEDS

How much information is necessary before preventive interventions can be designed and implemented is a matter of some disagreement (e.g., Albee 1982; Lorion, Price, and Eaton 1989). Elsewhere (Lorion 1990; Lorion, Price, and Eaton 1989) we have argued that the design and evaluation of interventions to prevent or treat emotional and behavioral disorders in children must be based on a thorough understanding of the developmental processes underlying those disorders. In the case of pervasive community violence, it is likely that complex transactional mechanisms involving individual and environmental factors (Lorion 1990; Sameroff and Fiese 1989) will need to be understood.

Completing the sequence from preliminary descriptive epidemiology to refining a promising intervention that can survive within the effected neighborhoods and be disseminated elsewhere will take considerable time (Price and Lorion 1989). Optimistically, a reasonable program of research on the effects of community violence on children could require a decade or more of preparatory work before viable solutions are widely available. Given that death and injury operationalize significant experimental measures within the line of inquiry, such caution seems ethically justified. It also seems ethically and socially unacceptable!

Can we as social and behavioral researchers genuinely ask communities to cooperate in the necessary research and to accept that little may change for at least a decade? Can we ask them to abandon one and maybe two generations of their children until we are certain? In return, will we commit ourselves to continuing involvement throughout whatever period of time is necessary? Will we do so without contingencies to that commitment such as "assuming the availability of funds" and "as long as I am on the faculty at . . . ?" In effect, will we enter into a partnership with participating communities in which *they* but *not we* have the option to terminate the partnership?

Our colleagues in the community raised such issues. From their perspective, collaboration involves more than *their* cooperating with the design and conduct of *our* data collection. Given *their* responsibilities, it also means that *we* are expected to assist them in determining the immediate and practical implications of the findings for program development and resource utilization. They recognize that doing so dilutes the "purity" of experimental designs. For them, however, scientific rigor must be balanced with social responsibility. In their view, evidence of *our* willingness to collaborate is reflected in our appreciation of the value of *their* priorities and of *their* perspectives.

Their comments have changed our sense of the minimum knowledge necessary for designing an "informed" intervention. As an alternative, systematic evaluations will be incorporated within initial efforts at interventions. This compromise offers a vehicle for both responding to critical needs and expanding the knowledge base necessary for ever-more refined interventions.

Acknowledging our admonitions about the need for further research, school, and community officials asked that we join with them immediately to design interventions for children from such neighborhoods. In response to media coverage of local events and our preliminary findings, the County Executive's Office committed significant funds to after-school programs, increased police patrols in high-risk neighborhoods, expanded play areas in such settings, and contributed to provision of in-service training for school personnel in crisis intervention. Federal and state funds have been obtained to design, implement, and evaluate interventions within some of the most dangerous neighborhoods.

FINAL COMMENT

Have we abandoned our commitment to scientific rigor? To some degree, yes! Methodological controls will be less than ideal; independent variables will be less firmly operationalized than desired. Community leaders and residents will participate in planning steps in the investigation and serve as an additional level of review for informed consent procedures. They will also extend our interpretations of findings and highlight paths to follow that we may have ignored. Hopefully, the scientific import of what we find will be confirmed through replication and cross-validation. At the very last, we expect that the ecological validity of our work will be significantly enhanced.

REFERENCES

ALBEE, G. W. Preventing psychopathology and promoting human potential. *American Psychologist* (1982) 37:1043-50.

BARKER, R. G. *Habitats, Environments, and Human Behavior.* Jossey-Bass, 1978.

BELL, C. C., and JENKINS, E. J. *Community violence and children on Chicago's Southside.* Unpublished manuscript, Community Mental Health Council, Chicago, 1990.

BRONFENBRENNER, V. Toward an experimental ecology of human development. *American Psychologist* (1977) 32:513-31.

DENNIS, R. E., KIRK, A., and KNUCKLES, B. N. *Black Males at Risk to Low Life Expectancy: A Study of Homicide Victims and Perpetrators.* National Institute of Mental Health, Center for Studies of Minority Group Mental Health, 1981.

DUBROW, N., and GARBARINO, J. Living in the war zone: Mothers and young children in a public housing development. *Child Welfare* (1989) 68(1):3-19.

EMDE, R. *Community violence exposure and emotional development.* Presentation made at conference: Community Violence and Childrens Development: Research and Clinical Implications, Washington, DC, November 16, 1990.

ERIKSON, E. H. *Childhood and Society.* W. W. Norton, 1963.

GARBARINO, J., KOSTELNY, K., and DUBROW, N. *Children and youth in dangerous environments: Coping with the consequences.* Unpublished manuscript, Erikson Institute for Advanced Study in Child Development, Chicago, 1989.

GARBARINO, J., KOSTELNY, K., and DUBROW, N. *No Place to Be a Child: Growing up in a War Zone.* Lexington Books, 1991.

GARBARINO, J., KOSTELNY, K., and DUBROW, N. *Children in Dangerous Environments: Coping with the Consequences of Community Violence.* Jossey-Bass, 1992.

GIBBS, J. T. Black adolescents and youth: An endangered species. *American Journal of Orthopsychiatry* (1984) 54(1):6-21.

HAWKINS, J. D., LISHNER, D., and CATALANO, R. F. Childhood predictors and the prevention of adolescent substance abuse. In C. L. Jones and R. J. Battles, eds., *Ethology of Drug Abuse: Implications for Prevention* (pp. 75-126). NIDA Research Monograph 56, DHHS Publ. No. (ADM) 85-1335. U.S. Government Printing Office, 1985.

JENKINS, E. J., and THOMPSON, B. *Children talk about violence: Preliminary findings from a survey of black elementary school children.* Paper presented at the 19th Annual Convention of the Association of Black Psychologists, Oakland, CA, 1986.

KOVAKS, M. The Children's Depression Inventory. *Psychopharmacology Bulletin* (1985) 21: 995-98.

LORION, R. P. Developmental analyses of community phenomena. In P. Tolan, C. Keys, F. Chertok, and L. Jason, eds., *Researching Community Psychology: Issues of Theory and Methods* (pp. 32-41). American Psychological Association, 1990.

LORION, R. P., BUSSELL, D., and GOLDBERG, R. Identification of youth at risk for alcohol or other drug problems. In E. N. Gopelrud, ed., *Preventing Adolescent Drug Use: From Theory to Practice.* (pp. 53-90) OSAP Prevention Monograph-8. DHHS Publ. No. (ADM) 90-1725. Office for Substance Abuse Prevention, 1991.

LORION, R. P., PRICE, R. H., and EATON, W. W. The prevention of child and adolescent disorders: From theory to research. In D. Shaffer, I. Phillips, and N. Enzer, eds., *Prevention of Mental Disorders, Alcohol and Other Drug Use in Children and Adolescents* (pp. 55-96). DHHS Publ. No. (ADM) 89-1646, Office of Substance Abuse Prevention, 1989.

MASLOW, A. *Motivation and Personality*, 2nd ed. Harper & Row, 1970.

NADER, K., PYNOOS, R., FAIRBANKS, L., and FREDERICK, C. *Childhood PTSD reactions in the year after a sniper attack.* Paper presented at the American Academy of Child and Adolescent Psychiatry, Beverly Hills, CA, 1988.

OSOFSKY, J. D., WEWERS, S., HANN, D. M., and FICK, A. C. Chronic community violence: What is happening to our children? *Psychiatry* (1993) 56: 36-45.

PRICE, R. H., and LORION, R. P. Prevention programming as organizational reinvention: From research to implementation. In D. Shaffer, I. Phillips, and N. Enzer, eds., *Prevention of Mental Disorders, Alcohol and Other Drug Use in Children and Adolescents* (pp. 97-124). DHHS Publ. No. (ADM) 89-1646. Office of Substance Abuse Prevention, 1989.

PYNOOS, R. S. The child as witness to homicide. *Journal of Social Issues* (1984) 40:87-108.

PYNOOS, R. S., and ETH, S. Children traumatized by witnessing acts of personal violence: Homicide, rape, and suicide behavior. In S. Eth and R. S. Pynoos, eds., *Post-traumatic Stress Disorder in Children.* (pp. 17-43). Washington, D.C.: American Psychiatric Press, 1985.

PYNOOS, R. S., FREDERICK, C., NADER, K., ARROYO, W., STEINBERG, A., ETH, S., NUNEZ, F., and FAIRBANKS, L. Life threat and posttraumatic stress in school-age children. *Archives of General Psychiatry* (1987) 44:1057–63

PYNOOS, R. S., and NADER, K. Children's memory and proximity to violence. *Journal of American Academy of Child and Adolescent Psychiatry* (1989) 28(2):236–41.

PYNOOS, R. S., and NADER, K. Psychological first aid and treatment approach to children exposed to community violence: research implications. *Journal of Traumatic Stress* (1988) 1(4):445–73.

RICHTERS, J. E., and MARTINEZ, P. *Checklist of Child Distress Symptoms: Parent Report.* National Institute of Mental Health, 1990.

RICHTERS, J. E., and SALTZMAN, W. R. *Survey of Children's Exposure to Community Violence: Parent Report.* National Institute of Mental Health, 1990.

RICHTERS, J. E., and MARTINEZ, P. The NIMH community violence project: I. Children as victims of and witnesses to violence. *Psychiatry* (1993) 56: 7–21.

RYAN, W. *Blaming the victim.* Random House, 1971.

RUBINETTI, F., and LORION, R. P. Gender, ethnicity, and drug use: Unexpected patterns in pre-adolescents.

SALTZMAN, W. *Children's exposure to violence.* Un-published master's thesis, University of Maryland, 1992.

SALTZMAN, W., and LORION, R. P. *Neighborhood risk and preadolescent drug use.* Presented at the Eastern Psychological Association, Philadelphia, PA, March 1990.

SAMEROFF, A. J., and FIESE, B. H. Conceptual issues in prevention. In S. Shaffer, I. Phillips, and N. B. Enzer, eds., *Prevention of Mental Disorders, Alcohol and Other Drug Use in Children and Adolescents* (pp. 7–22). DHHS Publ. No. (ADM) 89-1646, Office of Substance Abuse Prevention, 1989.

SARASON, S. B. If it can be studied or developed, should it be? *American Psychologist* (1984) 39: 477–85.

SHAKOOR, B. H., and CHALMERS, D. Co-victimization of African-American children who witness violence and the theoretical implications of its effects on their cognitive, emotional, and behavioral development. *Journal of the National Medical Association* (1991) 83(3):233–38.

SLAIKEU, K. A. *Crisis Intervention: A Handbook for Practice and Research.* Allyn and Bacon, 1990.

WICKER, W. *An Introduction to Ecological Psychology.* Brooks-Cole, 1979.

WILSON, W. *Thinking About Crime.* Basic Books, 1975.

Community Violence, Children's Development, and Mass Media: In Pursuit of New Insights, New Goals, and New Strategies

Bernard Z. Friedlander

Who will be hurt? Those who do not value the
life of a helpless child. . . . I'm going to hurt you
until you understand that the children are our
future and deserve to live. . . .
— M. C. Hammer, "Help the Children" (1990)

COMMUNITY VIOLENCE that victimizes children is an unmitigated evil
that is exacerbated by vast economic and social forces that leave people in central cities and the rural countryside adrift on seas of rolelessness, hopelessness,
group disintegration, and alienation. The contemporary drug scene and the
easy availability of guns greatly intensify violence on a local scale, while crimes
of violence, especially with guns, appear to be level or declining in the nation as
a whole. Claims that the persistently high levels of violence in mass media,
mostly television, are largely responsible for violence in society represent narrow views of very large issues. These narrow views overlook essential elements
of both phenomena—violence and media. Direct models of interpersonal violence in families and in the community probably give rise to more violent behavior than indirect models in media. Disinhibitory and provocative aspects of
media probably do as much or more to trigger violent behavior than violent narratives and violent actions. Comprehensive meta-analysis indicates that prosocial messages on television can have greater effects on behavior than antisocial
messages. These data support the contention that mass media can play a
strong and positive role in alleviating some of the distress of victims of community violence, and in redirecting the behavior of some of its perpetrators so as
to *protect the children*.

Bernard Z. Friedlander, PhD, is from the Department of Psychology, University of Hartford, West Hartford, CT 06117.
Send reprint requests to the author.
I would like to acknowledge the assistance of Peter Walsh of the Department of Biology, Yale University, for his assistance in helping me formulate the conceptual structure of the "cumulative precursor components of violent behavior," shown in Figure 1, and the editorial help of Julia Friedlander of the Stanford Law
School. I would also like to express my appreciation to Keith Cottam, Director, and the staff of the University of Wyoming library, who were so generous with their assistance and facilities during the summer of 1990
when I did the library research for this paper while teaching at the University of Wyoming, Laramie. William
Harris of Cambridge, MA, made valuable suggestions in the preparation of this manuscript for publication.

This paper is presented in six sections:

INTRODUCTION: FRAMING THE ISSUES

Early in my studies and my thought on community violence, children's development and mass media, I made the judgment that it is important to include ideas about *causation and prevention* as well as ideas about research and treating the effects of community violence on children. *Reducing both the incidence and the impact* of community violence to which children are exposed could be just as important as learning more about the developmental dysfunctions that stem from it and how these dysfunctions can be treated.

I also formed the opinion that it would not be a sufficient response to the present challenge simply to review what has been done in the arena where thoughts about mass media and thoughts about children encounter each other. In the center ring of this arena is the 30-year history of research on the effects of television violence on children's social behavior. For reasons that will become apparent, I found it necessary to seek fresh insights on relationships among the realities of community violence, the realities of children's development, and the realities of mass media in contemporary American life.

In my exploration of these realities, I came to see a very big problem with the existing research on television and children's social behavior. This big problem has nothing to do with internal questions of whether this research is good research, or whether its claims are true.

The big problem is the external one. For 30 years research on the effects of television on children and on their social behavior has had generous funds, generous opportunities, and an exceptionally high degree of penetration into the corridors of power. Yet this research, for whatever reason, has had no meaningful impact on the levels of violence in media, no impact on practices in the media industries, and no impact on child-rearing practices in the vast majority of American households in our media-dominated world.

The recently passed federal Children's Television Act of 1989 is a case in point (U.S. Congress 1990). It represents years of exhausting political advocacy. Yet all it does is trim a few minutes per hour and some of the grosser exploitations from the barrage of advertising on broadcast television programming directed toward children. And within 3 weeks of its passage, FCC attorneys were bogged down in the problem of enforcing it without wounding the commercial side of the Sesame Street operation—no one wants to hinder the marketing of dolls and toys whose revenues help sustain the high costs of the Sesame Street television programs (*Hartford Courant* 1990).

On the specific issue of violence, nothing has changed. There is a dismal consistency in Gerbner's data on high levels of violence in television from 1967 to 1985. Gerbner's data show that, if anything, *television programs became more rather than less violent*—during the very period when concern about media violence was at the highest tide of its public visibility (Gerbner, Gross, Signorielli, and Morgan 1986). This example of high profile ineffectuality suggests that strategic reconsideration would be in order for those willing to learn from this lesson.

As I found out more about the pervasiveness, the intensity, and the destructiveness of community violence in its impact on children's lives, it became increasingly apparent to me that there was little or nothing to be gained by pursuing the old debates that have dominated the frontline research on television and social behavior. There was nothing to be gained by falling into the same pattern of conspicuous impotence. If there were to be hope for progress and useful change, it would be necessary to pursue new goals and new strategies. It would be necessary to pursue pathways toward social change for which research may be an instrument of progress and not simply a goal in and of itself.

From my vantage point, four sets of meaningful outcomes of studying community violence and children's development appear to be both desirable and attainable. The first task is to examine children's experience with violence as a specific and distinctively potent *developmental disorganizer* in the course of their psychological growth. As noted below, it is urgent to gain more detailed knowledge on the proposition that violence in childhood plays an especially destructive part in setting children on the path toward pain-filled lives of school failure, unemployability, dependency, and pervasive dysfunctionality.

Second, we must assemble first-class epidemiological data on community violence similar to the Straus and Gelles work on family violence (Straus and Gelles 1990). Their success in identifying and publicizing previously unrecognized details of family violence shows how important it is to have a hard data platform when formulating goals and evaluating long-term change.

Third, we need a clearer view of an "ecology of violence" than we presently possess, and we need to learn more about how mass media fit in with other individual and situational factors that give rise to the violent behavior in the community to which children are exposed.

The fourth task is to seek and pursue practical measures to *protect the children* from community violence that does occur.

In terms of raw reality, present levels of violence are not likely to be reduced over the short term due to the deep structure of intractable social forces from which this violence springs. This reality entails extending the concept of *protecting children* to a concept of *reducing the incidence of violence* in settings where children have a right to be without having to be afraid of harm.

It is at this juncture that it seems both practical and attainable to seek a positive role for mass media commensurate with the media's capacity to exert great social leverage. Framing the issue in these terms requires a switch by child advocates from persisting in a Cold War mentality that sees media only as the inevitable demon adversary.

Lest this seem like an odd twist in the path of child advocacy, we only need to look about us to see evidence to justify optimism that *there can be progress and improvement* in national social problems and world-level confrontations that are no less destructive than inflicting violence upon defenseless children. Examples abound: the end of the Cold War, the start on dismantling apartheid, the rise of environmentalism, the expansion of gender parity, and the stigmatization of cigarette smoking. Who among us who struggled alone against the tide to stop smoking 30 years ago could have imagined that we would live to see the era of the smoke-free office building in which it is the smokers who are in the defensive minority?

In 1973 when Straus presented his first theoretical formulation on violence in families (Straus 1973), it probably did not seem plausible that he and his associates would be able to report discernible reductions in family violence less than 20 years later (Reardon 1990).

These numerous signs that positive change can take place, even in the most intricate and recalcitrant social problems, suggest that a glimmer of optimism may not be entirely out of place in our concern for children's development in settings of traumatic community violence.

PLACING VIOLENCE AT THE TOP OF THE LIST OF SOCIAL EVILS THAT DEBASE CHILDHOOD

Violence

In her comprehensive analysis of social disorganization and means to combat it, Lisbeth Schorr (1989, p. 3) places violence and violent crime right at the top of the list of reversible societal, familial, and individual disorders that combine to produce the downward spiral of decay she terms "the high cost rotten outcomes" of broken lives among the modern American poor. Along with violence and crime go the other disorders that are parts of a familiar picture: school-age pregnancy, dropping out of school, unemployability, and households headed by impoverished single women.

Schorr reminds us that where violence and crime are endemic, virtually everyone in the affected communities participates in them—as victims, as witnesses, and/or as perpetrators. We have singled out children for our special attention because we think they should be and perhaps can be protected in some special category. Until the children gain some special protected status, they are part of the violence and crime that define the everyday structure of their communities. As things stand now, the children's lives are tightly woven into the fabric of organization or disorganization of their community's grinding, impoverished struggle for competitive survival that is one of its outstanding characteristics.

The struggle is compounded by the "four horsemen" of a new apocalypse: rolelessness, hopelessness, group disintegration, and alienation (Foster 1990; Nightingale and Wolverton 1988). The facts of violence and crime are as fundamental in this fabric of personal and interpersonal behavior as are deindustrialization of the workforce, the flight of employment due to the internationalization of the economy, and the resulting decapitalization of urban neighborhoods and the rural countryside. Where systemic poverty prevails, victimized children are participants in the international economy who suffer all its downside hazards and gain few of its upside benefits.

It is a fundamental error to fail to take these macrosystem elements into account when trying to understand the basic structure of the problem of community violence as it affects children.

Children's Development

There are several reasons why community violence affecting children is so clearly an unmitigated evil. One reason is the children's helpless vulnerability. It is just unbearably *unfair* that children who cannot protect themselves are targeted and exploited as intended or unintended victims.

Another reason we professionals see the full face of evil when children are victims of violence is because we are just beginning to understand its devastating developmental impact. Except for the rare individuals who have some special stamina or resilience, we have come to see that violence is cruelly damaging to the essential roots of children's growth toward competent adulthood.

Just as violence and crime are elemental parts of the structure of life where they are endemic, trust and security in durable personal attachments are elemental requirements for a decent life in any present and for any future. Whether we are guided by Erikson, by Bowlby, by Maslow, or any other theorist with comparable breadth, the compelling need for basic trust and reliable support in learning to cope with fear is at the psychological foundation of healthy humanity. When we try to nurture children's developmental opportunities, we try to enhance trust and cultivate secure attachments. There can be no more diabolical way to degrade children's developmental opportunities than to allow violence to undermine their trust, their security, and their attachments, and to infect them with unresolvable fear (Tuan 1979).

In these terms, we can see that the major developmental damage caused to the greatest number of children by community violence is not that it makes them become violent as they grow up—as is commonly and erroneously supposed. (Note Widom reference in the section on identification of precursors.) There is a bigger problem, both to individuals and to society. Children who are wounded by chronic violence trauma are likely to grow up impaired in their capacity to attain adaptive competence in their personal autonomy, their educational performance, their employability, their citizenship, and their ability to maintain effective interpersonal relationships.

Mass Media

Mass media are as elemental in the structure of modern American life as violence and crime are elemental in life wherever it occurs, as trust and security are elemental in healthy psychological development, and as violence and fear are elemental in putting healthy development at risk. Whenever we consider a topic of which mass media are a component, we must bear in mind that the media—principally but not exclusively television—have redefined some of the most tradition-bound aspects of American society since the onset of the electronic revolution after World War II. The media have redefined politics and the electoral system, they have redefined church membership, they have redefined entertainment, they have redefined baseball, and some astute observers say they have redefined childhood (Meyrowitz 1985; Postman 1981).

It is a mistake to think of video as simply another source of particular kinds of messages. The essence of video is its virtual universality, its virtually universal accessibility, and its irreversible absorption into the basic rituals of daily life (Kubey & Csikszentmihalyi 1990). Almost anybody almost anywhere can see and hear almost anything at almost any time. For example, it is naive and old-fashioned to think that we can somehow control children's exposure to violence on television by challenging the First Amendment to try to regulate program content on network broadcasting—in an age when video cable and videocassettes are devouring the broadcast audience.

One of the many reasons why the video age puts so much stress on childhood and family relationships is the difficulty it creates for even the most conscientious full-time parents to act as intermediaries between children and the outside world. Historically, this is one of the most important functions of parenthood—to protect children from the full weight of the adult world and to filter their knowledge of it. This is an exceptionally difficult assignment in the best of times and the best of circumstances.

This kind of protection and filtering is virtually impossible in our media world in households under the additional assaults of poverty and community disorganization. We must proceed under the ecological recognition that the children who are victimized by violence, as well as the youths and adults whose violent behavior torments them, are all equally embedded in their mass media biosphere as thoroughly as fish in a river are embedded in the water that surrounds them.

Embeddedness in the ecology of media can lead to outcomes for which we are not fully prepared. Let me cite two examples: first, the violence on television may be less immediate, less dangerous, and less terrifying than the violence on the street or in the family. Children are actually safer watching television mayhem in which the stray bullets are contained within the video tube than they are out on the street or in an armed family brawl where the bullets are real—and can kill. Second, in his brilliant ethnographic description of the youth drug trade in New Haven, Connecticut, Finnegan reports that the youths he observed were sometimes motivated and rewarded in their violent behavior by the prospect of having their arrests reported on the evening television news. They gained status in their peer group and among their girlfriends by having their names and their exploits described by television anchors, and by being seen on television as they were led off in handcuffs by police (Finnegan 1990).

As far as I am aware, there is nothing in the vast body of research on television violence and children's social behavior that can lay a finger on these levels of reality.

LOCUS AND FOCUS OF THE COMMUNITY VIOLENCE PROBLEM

It is very important to find out where the community violence problem is, how long it's been going on, and who is involved in it. We generally assume that the minority ethnic enclaves in the centers of our rotting cities are the principal settings of community violence, and that it is a recent phenomenon. Several observations suggest that this assumption might better be viewed as a hypothesis rather than as an axiom. The assumption is based largely on the frequently reported experiences of people who live and/or work in those settings, and on high-impact media reports of murderous horrors that recur in these urban settings with depressing frequency.

Contradicting the assumption of recency, there is ample evidence that the extremely violent nature of American community and family life that affects children is a deeply historical phenomenon (Gordon 1988; Graham and Gurr 1969; Straus, Gelles, and Steinmetz 1980). Brutalization of children is a recurrent theme in the legendary violence of our remote as well as our recent past (Campbell 1990). In some settings the children have been incidental bystanders or victims of adult-to-adult guns, knives, or eye-gougings, and comparable assaults. In other settings they have been the targeted objects of individual acts of sadism as well as of vicious group exploitation — such as child labor in mines, mills, factories, and on the farm.

It is also sadly true that the rural countryside can be as hazardous for children as the urban slum. I discovered this by direct encounter during the summer of 1990, when I taught a workshop on developmental psychology to a group of experienced educators at the University of Wyoming. Wyoming is perhaps the most rural and "whitest" of all 50 states in the Union, and it claims the reputation of having the highest per capita rate in the country for unwed school-age pregnancies.

I was appalled at the frequency with which my informants reported the plight of children in remote communities far out in the thinly populated countryside who were trapped in settings dominated by assaultive and murderous clan conflicts, feuds, property disputes, political antagonisms, brutal and often alcoholic families, vehicular homicides, and suicides.

We should keep these rural children well in mind. There may be hundreds of thousands, or perhaps millions, of children exposed to community violence in the cities, but there are surely tens of thousands suffering the same fate in the countryside. On an individual basis, the pain, the destruction, and the need for protective intervention for the country children are just as great as for those in the cities.

The scope, the precision, and the data of the National Family Violence Surveys described by Straus and Gelles (1990) point to the indispensable value of the sort of baseline data that is needed in the realm of community violence. Until some semblance of this sort of data is compiled, it will be difficult to determine with any exactitude the different causes and forms of violence for which different forms of intervention are required, and where and by whom these interventions are needed. Without such determinations, it will be impossible to establish a rational basis for directing aid to the children who need it most.

We cannot forecast exactly what these data will reveal but we can expect that they will produce surprises. For example, without the Straus and Gelles data on family violence, who would have expected that the incidence of severe violence against children is higher from older siblings than from parents? (1990, p. 97). As they become assembled, data on community violence are almost certain to produce comparable surprises.

COMMUNITY VIOLENCE AS CRIME

Violence trauma that is so hurtful to children who are afflicted by it is almost always an outcome of criminal behavior. Child advocates and mental health professionals tend to overlook the criminal nature of the physical and psychological assaults that community violence inflicts upon children. This criminal behavior is just as much in the domain of the criminal justice system as it is in the domain of the mental health professions. When children or their siblings, parents, friends, and neighbors are terrified and unwilling witnesses or direct victims of guns and gunshot wounds, knifings, beatings, physical assaults, forced entries, muggings, robberies, and rapes, they are in the grip of overtly criminal acts.

In his analysis of family violence, Emery (1989) contends that "those professionals who are . . . responsible for intervention are encouraged to use definitions and responses to family violence that match those used for assaults between strangers"—namely by invoking the criminal justice system. The same generalization is just as applicable to community violence. The fact that the criminal justice system and the system of jails and prisons have poor records in dealing with roots of crime doesn't mean we should call crime by some other name.

As we learn more about the demographics of community violence and come to regard it as the pattern of criminal behavior that it really is, we will learn to differentiate between the *prevalence* and the *incidence* of violent crime. This is a crucial distinction made by eminent researchers in the fields of criminology and criminal justice, and it is a distinction the mental health professions, the media, legislatures, the ordinary public, and even many among the police generally do not understand. Elliott, Huizinga and other national leaders in this field (Elliott 1989; El-

liott, Huizinga, and Menard 1989) point to the crucial importance of distinguishing between the proportion of the population involved in criminal activity, which is *prevalence*; and the frequency of occurrence of criminal activity, which is *incidence*.

In their powerful analyses, it is apparent that the *prevalence* of crime in the United States ("who does it") is level or perhaps even declining. Increasing *incidence* of crime ("how much do they do") can be seen in the rising frequency and intensity of crime due to two special factors that are highly relevant to our concern for ascertaining the locus and the focus of community violence. First, the increasing use of guns in controversies over turf in the drug trade increases the severity of violence, as seen in the phenomenon of seemingly casual shootings of adversaries and of innocent bystanders. (We should remember that Mercutio and Tybalt in *Romeo and Juliet* were slain in the 14th-century Veronese equivalent of drive-by shootings—for flimsier reasons than drug deals gone sour. Maybe neither would have died if they had had real jobs and were working at them, instead of roaming the streets, looking for trouble and finding it.)

Second, Elliott (1989) makes the especially important point that the increasing incidence of crime is due largely to the fact that social changes such as structural unemployment, related to vast economic change and the decapitalization of neighborhoods as already noted, tend to perpetuate the length and recidivism of individual criminal careers in settings where there is no adequately absorptive job market into which crime-prone juveniles can "graduate" when they enter adulthood.

Other authoritative statistical analyses of firearms use and firearms offenses point in the same direction. Kleck (1989a) maintains that we are actually experiencing a *decline* in the prevalence of criminal offenses involving firearms. Horrifying firearms offenses like the Stockton, California, hate crime schoolyard massacre of Asian children and the casual, routine frequency of shootings in the street get high visibility play in mass media news. These reports give the impression that the prevalence of criminal offenses involving firearms has gone upward. But Kleck claims the reverse is true, maintaining that solid data uphold his view that "the assault rifle problem [is] largely a media creation" (1989b).

The mass media tend to focus their attention – and the attention of the public, the legislatures, and even the police – on highly conspicuous individual incidents and not upon broadly based and very intricate statistical trends. Thus it is easy to understand how misapprehensions gain very wide currency, and there is a tendency for these misapprehensions to guide public opinion, professional discourse, and legislative action. This tendency makes it even more important that the professional groups whose job it is to repair and prevent the damage of social carnage where it does occur should have a clear and fact-based understanding of the issues as they actually exist.

IDENTIFYING PRECURSOR COMPONENTS OF VIOLENT BEHAVIOR

Background

Some of the frontline research on television violence and social behavior is exceptionally powerful. In the introductory chapter to their book *Television and the Aggressive Child*, Huesmann and Eron (1986a) make a very persuasive case that television violence does indeed prompt some aggression-prone youths to be more aggressive and violent than they would otherwise be without it. Conceptualizing aggression as a precursor to violence, their analysis is very astute. It goes far beyond the notion that a single source of influence can account for aggressive and violent behavior. Succinctly surveying a large body of behavioral and social research, they point out that:

The truth is . . . no one factor by itself predicts aggressiveness very well. . . . The innate aggressive responses one finds in lower animals cannot usually be demonstrated in humans . . . [and] the mounting evidence suggests that aggression is to a great extent learned. For most children, aggressiveness seems to be determined mostly by the extent to which their environment reinforces aggression, provides aggressive models, frustrates and victimizes the child, and instigates aggression. Thus, *to understand the development of aggression, one must examine simultaneously a multiplicity of interrelated social, cultural, familial and cognitive factors, each of which adds only a small increment to the totality of causation. It is unrealistic to expect that any one of these factors by itself can explain much about aggression. But in conjunction with each other they may explain a lot about aggression.* [emphasis added] (p. 4)

This passage tells us how essential it is to look beyond any single factor as the provocation, cause, or explanation for violence in the community. This is not a lesson that is generally understood by many of the professionals and lay people who seem to regard television and other mass media as the principal explanation for high levels of violence in the community and in the lives of children – the vector they hold to be most deserving of intense scrutiny and regulatory intervention.

The multicausal nature of aggression and violence seems as obvious as Huesmann and Eron claim it to be. Yet a great deal of academic energy has been devoted to a prosecutorial fixation on getting a conviction against television as the most culpable of all prospective suspects – without making equally energetic investigations or prosecutions of other, possibly more culpable, suspects (Levinger et al., 1986). This view also leads to elaborate technofixes when the data on television and antisocial behavior show only small effects (Rosenthal 1986). Meanwhile, other suspects on the charge of committing acts of violence trauma against children roam at large, and only the mass media are expected to take the heat.

Foreground

Reiss (1986) points out the very practical and useful lesson that *segregating the variance* is the first requirement when we bring together information from several disciplines to try to solve a common problem. Perhaps we can apply that lesson in seeking an enhanced understanding of how violence in the community occurs, so that we could then go on to Reiss's second requirement for integrating knowledge, which is the detailed *clarification of mechanisms*.

It helps to think of any individual or group act or sequence of acts of violence as a behavioral summation of multiple components. Each of these components is present and operative at some variable level of intensity before the violence occurs. Whether the target is a person or an object of property, and whether the violence is committed by a single person or a group, the components are likely to be the same, even though they may be combined in different ways in different settings, with different perpetrators and with different victims.

Threshold   * * * * *Z:* Violent Behavior * * * *

Y: Releaser or disinhibitor
(e.g., alcohol, drugs, anger, rage, crowd or gang effect, or subjective imagery)

X: Provocation or incentive
(e.g., sexual challenge; personal or group challenge to esteem; gang rivalry; ethnic rivalry; interpersonal quarrel; craving for possession, power, or control; territoriality, "target of opportunity")

W: Contextual Constellation
(e.g., possession of weapon, changing patterns of police surveillance)

↑
Situational Factors
Individual Factors
↓

V: Disregard for consequences
(e.g., defiance of detection or punishment)

U: Direct behavioral models
(e.g., in the family, among peers, in the neighborhood)

T: Indirect behavioral models
(e.g., images in videos, comic books, movies, pop music, etc.)

S: Personal history
(e.g., victimization, frustration, reinforcement of prior aggression and violence)

R: Personality
(e.g., decompensated ego structure; impulsive, risk-taking temperament)

Figure 1.
Cumulative precursor components of violent behavior.

Let us think of violent behavior as Z at the end of the line – above a flashpoint threshold of activation. Then the precursor components work backward in a rough approximation of ordinality like this:

Y – a releaser or disinhibitor (e.g., alcohol, drugs, anger, rage, crowd or gang effect, subjective imagery)

X – a provocation or incentive (e.g., sexual challenge, personal or group challenge to esteem, gang rivalry, ethnic rivalry, interpersonal quarrel, craving for possession, power or control, "target of opportunity")

W – an interpersonal or contextual constellation of circumstances (e.g., possession of weapon, changes in police surveillance)

V – disregard for consequences (e.g., defiance of detection or punishment)

U – direct behavioral models (e.g., in the family, among peers, in the neighborhood)

T – indirect behavioral models (e.g., images in video, comic books, movies, pop music, etc).

S – personal history (e.g., victimization, frustration, reinforcement of prior aggression and violence)

R – personality (e.g., decompensated ego structure, impulsive, risk-taking temperament)

According to this ordinal-sequential model of violence, as shown in Figure 1, "segments of the variance" that are close to the threshold of activation are more likely to be specifically *situational* triggering factors, varying in likelihood of occurrence from moment to moment and from setting to setting. Those components further from the threshold are more likely to be generalized and ongoing *individual* factors in shaping the likelihood of violence – necessary but not sufficient in themselves for the explosion of violent behavior to occur.

What is most notable about this sequential hierarchy is that the indirect models of violent behavior as seen in mass media are so far from the threshold where the trouble bursts forth. No thoughtful person who knows the research literature would deny that scenes of violence seen repeatedly on television by children and other people might have something to do with generating the reality of violence in their behavior. But in the light of the other factors at work that also contribute to the total, the component of indirect behavior modeling from media imagery is unlikely to have the preemptive importance that has been attributed to it.

If there is a body of research that seeks to assess the relative weight of the mass media component in the context of other, identified situational and individual components in the expression of aggressive and violent behavior, I have not been able to find it.

The way this model differentiates situational from individual factors in the cumulative hierarchy also helps to explain why many individuals – undoubtedly the vast majority – who are exposed to high levels of violence in life and in media *do not* commit acts of violence in their own behavior. This phenomenon is at the root of a recent major challenge to the concept of "the cycle of violence." Widom's cohort study found that "being abused or neglected as a child increases one's risk of delinquency, adult criminal behavior, and violent criminal behavior. However the majority of abused and neglected children do not become delinquent, criminal or violent" (Widom 1989). It is essential to note that this finding says nothing about neglect, abuse, and violence as developmental precursors of victimization and dysfunctionality.

Nothing in this intricate web of relationships suggests that television's instrumental role in the problem of community violence is negligible. In fact, there are two other "segments of the variance" – right at the flashpoint threshold at the top of the hierarchy – where mass media influence, and especially television, may be closer to the action than has been recognized. The first of these is the component involving *release of violence and disinhibition of behavioral control*. The second is the component involving *provocation to violence* in any of the listed categories—provocations that may range from challenges against personal or group esteem to craving for power or possession of objects. These components are represented in media with exceptionally high intensity and exceptionally high redundancy in the media lifestyle of affluent materialism and in the imagery of power and control portrayed by media heroes.

It is plausible to maintain that the factor of *addictive disinhibition* is one of the most fundamental elements in the operating realities of mass media, most especially commercial television, where the principal objective of entertainment programs and advertising is to overcome whatever inhibitions might deter the viewer from watching the programs and buying the products. In this respect, mass media contribute mightily to a culture of disinhibition. Television does not set out to cultivate violence but to cultivate disinhibited behavior. Violence is simply one of the ways in which the disinhibition and disregard of internalized behavioral restraints manifest themselves.

Finnegan (1990) portrays these elements at work with chilling power in the violence of the urban drug scene in his recent ethnographic descriptive masterpiece: "A Street Kid in the Drug Trade." Finnegan paints a catastrophic picture—like a Heironymous Bosch altarpiece—of a world and its inhabitants fallen apart, or never having had the chance to get put together. Violent drug and gang affiliations, both inside the school and outside it among the school dropouts, provide virtually the only option for even temporary personal safety among youths ungifted in school skills who struggle against being wiped out in an urban jungle.

In addition to the constant, violent, competitive battling for identity, prestige, and dominance within the gang and between the gangs that Finnegan describes, the struggle is complicated and intensified by a profoundly rooted "ideology" of consumer individualism "imbibed since childhood from commercial television" as a belief system, a kind of secular religion. When this consumerist belief system collides with the transgenerational poverty and hopelessness associated with structural unemployment, school failure, and virtual unemployability, the violent affiliative network of gang membership and the lucrative drug trade offers itself as the only apparent path of escape from a desperate life. The vivid, continuous, exquisitely seductive, and high-energy mass media imagery of abandoned impulsivity and disinhibition combines with equally vivid, equally continuous, and equally seductive mass media imagery of effortless affluence. When these floods of images engulf energetic youths and young adults trapped on islands of poverty and hopelessness, it should be no surprise that the consequences take the form of seemingly pervasive acts of violence.

Investigators and commentators who gaze obsessively at television violence as if it were the paramount cause of behavioral violence are probably looking in the wrong direction with only a single eye—seeing only the symptomatic rash on the surface, and not the immunochemical struggle taking place within. It is much more fruitful to look at the complexity of the media biosphere and the complexity of violent behavior within that biosphere in order to find ways to have some practical, limiting effects on the catastrophic violent behavior we want to try to change.

In terms of the framework of precursor components presented here as a way to think about violent behavior, there is room to disagree on details about how the deep structure of explosive forces within individuals interacts with the surface structure of situational triggers, thus leading to outbreaks of community violence that traumatize children. But these ideas can serve as a useful means to move forward beyond the limitations of current models and current data of social-learning research. That research may meet the criteria of scientific method, but it does not deal adequately with the complexity of the phenomena it studies, and it has had little or no social utility in dealing effectively with an increasingly disastrous blight on the lives of large numbers of children.

MOVING TOWARD PRACTICAL ACTION: FINDING A POSITIVE ROLE FOR MASS MEDIA

If community violence that traumatizes children is the visible symptom of the deeper disorders of poverty, international economics, structural unemployment, rolelessness, and group disorganization, then it is probable that the most effective and thoroughgoing way to relieve the symptoms is to treat the underlying causes. But a strategy for doing that is not within the jurisdiction or the skills of the mental health and human development professionals who make up this constituency. Furthermore, we would be copping out of our responsibility to the children who are being wounded by community violence today, tomorrow, and next week if help for them were to be contingent on our nation's ability to solve some of its most fundamental economic and social problems. If there is to be action, the action should start *now*, not on some happy day when we get to the other side of a rainbow.

Of course, this action should include the obvious things such as strengthening neighborhood clinics, family support systems, community social services, and child protection programs in the schools. The success or failure of these actions will be shaped by the same factors of energy, competence, and availability of funds that determine the outcome of any social intervention program. Like virtually all social intervention programs, the supply of services will never be sufficient to meet the need and the demand. Poised as we are amid the economic debris of the 1980s and the uncertainties of a deepening recession, the gap is likely to widen rather than diminish between the supply and the need for social intervention services affecting children.

Part of the need and part of the demand for relief from the trauma of community violence can be expressed in terms of providing services to individual children and individual families. Even in the best of times there is a finite limit to the number of persons who can be served on an individual case-by-case basis, in terms of available funds and available personnel. In times of downward budgetary spirals, such as now and in the foreseeable future, that limit is likely to be lower than in the past.

Another part of the need and demand for relief from the trauma of community violence can be expressed in terms of public information, public opinion, and public sentiments about the special needs and vulnerabilities of children and childhood. This is an altogether different domain, and it is a domain where the mass media can play a highly instrumental role in reaching very large numbers of people—including the children who are most at risk of suffering from and the youths and adults who are most likely to perpetrate the damage of community violence.

With this second category of needs and demands in mind, I am proposing a major, long-term, highly sophisticated professional media campaign to promote many themes and actions that have the single purpose of protecting and being decent to children. On the positive side, I am proposing that the campaign have the professionalism, the identity, the persistence, and the purpose of protecting children against harm that Smokey Bear has had for almost 50 years in raising the national consciousness about the need to protect trees from forest fires (McNamara, Kurth, and Hansen 1989). Also on the positive side, I am proposing strategies that have the high penetration of the McGruff "Take a Bite out of Crime" campaign. This campaign reached approximately 50% of its intended audience—an astonishingly successful result (O'Keefe and Reid 1989). These campaigns have had the advantage of being generated and supervised almost exclusively by professional advertising and media personnel.

On the negative side, I am *not* proposing replication of the well-intentioned but brief and inconclusive ad hoc health and health-related campaigns summarized in the NIMH volumes edited by Pearl, Bouthilet, and Lazar (1982). These campaigns had the disadvantage of being generated and supervised mainly by academics and medical personnel closely associated with the health and health-related issues that were the subject of the campaigns. Also on the negative side, it is important to acknowledge McGuire's (1986) minimal effects analyses of media impacts, without being disabled by them.

This is no setting in which to engage in controversy over media methods, but it is essential to stress that the child protection campaigns I envisage would have the same driven intensity, the same mastery of media demographics and technology, and the same mobilization of celebrities, talent, energy, and art as such campaigns as the "Revolution" and "Just Do It" campaigns that more than doubled the sale of NIKE shoes (Berger 1990). To be successful, the child protection campaigns would also have to shift styles between the kindest, lightest touch of a baby soap product ad and the bizarre appeal to their intended audience of Madonna's 1990 flag-draped "Vote" campaign or the utterly manic Defense of the First Amendment segment of the 1990 Music Television Awards ceremony.

These are appeals that most intellectuals and professional people unfamiliar with studies of popular culture and unfamiliar with the media industries can neither comprehend, account for, nor explain. These aspects of modern media are like the cave paintings and petroglyphs of our prehistoric ancestors: They communicate with and provide insights about the minds of the people to whom they are important, but they require very special sensitivities and very special training to be understood by outsiders who function on different wavelengths of meaning.

Furthermore, the campaign would be planned to go on year after year after year—like Smokey Bear and Sesame Street. And like Smokey Bear and Sesame Street, the campaigns would be conducted by media professionals, not by subject-matter professionals. Finally, after initial start-up funding by a media-savvy foundation (like the MacArthur Foundation) and extremely careful selection of a highly committed directorate, I forecast that the ongoing campaign would do turnaway business in receiving personal and corporate subsidies and volunteer talent from every direction to keep it going. High-level media authorities with whom I have discussed this matter agree that voluntary participation and support would be very substantial if the project got off to a good start.

All this would be in the service of two principal goals:[1]

1. To reach children who are high-risk targets of violence with carefully crafted, high-redundancy messages that the children are needed, wanted, and cherished—and that they can be protected from harm by special link-up programs in their schools and neighborhood agencies, identified by symbols that in time would gain the same high recognition as Big Bird and Smokey Bear.
2. To reach perpetrators of violence with carefully crafted, high-redundancy messages that the children are needed, wanted, and cherished—*and that it is definitely uncool to mess them up*. Whatever else they do, they should *protect the children* or at least leave them alone.

In the last 30 years our nation has made dramatic if inadequate progress in dealing with immensely complicated problems such as environmental pollution, auto safety, voting rights, education and community access for the disabled, and reduced consumption of alcohol, tobacco, and drugs. But we're doing a rotten job of protecting the physical and psychological

---

[1]During the 8-week period between the time when this article was written and its revision for publication, M. C. Hammer's new rap, "Help the Children"—in the album *Please Hammer Don't Hurt 'Em*, with lyrics dealing with both these themes—began rising very high on the charts.

Table 1

EFFECT SIZES FOR TYPES OF ANTISOCIAL AND PROSOCIAL BEHAVIORS

	Average effect size[a]	SD	SE_M	No. of effects
Antisocial Behaviors				
Family discussion reduced	2.33	–	–	1
Role stereotyping	0.90	1.42	0.50	8
Less socialization	0.75	0.75	0.38	4
Rule breaking	0.56	0.65	0.17	14
Hurt (rather than help)	0.47	0.21	0.09	6
Materialism	0.40	0.83	0.16	26
Perception of world as violent	0.40	0.20	0.06	10
Playing with aggressive toys	0.37	0.59	0.22	7
Passivity	0.36	0.38	0.14	7
Physical aggression	0.31	0.80	0.05	229
Verbal and physical aggression	0.31	0.58	0.06	90
Perception of self as powerless	0.31	–	–	1
Willingness to use violence/ perceived as effective	0.27	0.39	0.09	21
Pathological behavior: nightmares, wets bed, louder	0.26	0.42	0.24	3
Negative attitude toward own culture	0.17	–	–	1
Unlawful behavior	0.13	0.41	0.09	20
Increased worry about the future	0.11	0.14	0.07	4
Use of drugs	0.09	0.33	0.11	9
Verbal aggression	0.05	0.41	0.10	17
Prosocial Behaviors				
Self-control	0.98	0.13	0.08	3
Altruism	0.83	1.18	0.20	36
Buy books	0.81	0.61	0.18	12
Mixture of socially desirable behaviors	0.78	1.12	0.50	5
Safety, health, and conservation activism	0.69	0.71	0.25	8
Positive attitude toward work	0.57	0.71	0.41	3
Antistereotyping; acceptance of others	0.57	0.61	0.14	2
Respect for the law	0.23	0.15	0.11	2
Play without aggression	0.21	–	–	1
Socially active/communicative	0.17	0.58	0.16	14
Creative, imaginative play	0.02	0.48	0.28	3
Cooperation	0	0.88	0.62	2

From: Hearold (1986).
[a]Reported effect sizes are based on the comparison of antisocial treatment versus other for antisocial behavior, and prosocial treatment versus other for prosocial behavior.

well-being of our most defenseless children. In many settings where they are most at risk, their needs are barely on the agenda of the people closest to them, who can give them the most help or do them the most harm.

I do not claim that the program I'm suggesting here can meet all their needs. But at least it can send the message that help is on the way, and it can give these children and the people around them a new awareness of the children's value, their importance to their communities, and their deservingness. And furthermore, the broad-based media campaigns I call for can accomplish these goals without legislation or the need for public sector funds.

CONCLUSION

In the entire professional literature that went into the preparation of this report, one page stands out as most relevant to conclude the presentation. This is the summary table from Hearold's (1986) meta-analysis of 1043 effects of television and social behavior. It is reprinted here as Table 1.

All that is necessary to do is to glance down the center column of this table and see that with a few exceptions, the effect sizes for prosocial media messages range higher than the effect sizes for antisocial media messages. It is not necessary to make a detailed study of these data to be persuaded that they point clearly to the

positive values that can be transmitted by television. Not only is it incomplete to regard television as a major or principal source of antisocial influences on behavior, it is wrong to assume that the antisocial messages propagated by television are necessarily more potent than the prosocial ones. In fact, potentially, it all may be the other way around.

These data lend great weight to the possibility that when properly mobilized, the full power of television and other mass media could play a major, long-term role in alleviating the intensity and the frequency of community violence trauma on children. They also lend weight to the possibility that this mobilization of mass media could contribute to a raising of the national consciousness and a long-term enhancement of our national commitment in family life, in education, and in all realms of our society that we must do a better job than we have been doing to *protect the children.*

One thing is sure: We will never know until we try.

REFERENCES

BARLOW, G., and HILL, A. *Video Violence and Children.* St. Martin's Press, 1985, pp. 160ff.

BELL, C. C., and JENKINS, E. J. Community violence and children on Chicago's Southside. *Psychiatry* (1993) 56:46–54.

BERGER, W. They know Bo. *New York Times Magazine,* November 11, 1990.

BRYANT, J., and ANDERSON, D. R. *Children's Understanding of Television: Research on Attention and Comprehension.* Academic Press, 1983, p. 152.

CAMPBELL, S. An end to years of closed doors, misread signs. *Hartford Courant,* October 29, 1990, p. B-1.

CATER, D., and STRICKLAND, S. *TV Violence and the Child: The Evolution and Fate of the Surgeon General's Report.* Russell Sage Foundation, 1975, pp. 10, 13, 50, 52, 75, 83.

DORR, A. *Television and Children: A Special Medium for a Special Audience.* Sage, 1986.

ELLIOTT, D. S. Testimony and prepared statement before U.S. House of Representatives Select Committee on Children, Youth, and Families, Washington, DC, May 16, 1989.

ELLIOTT, D. S., HUIZINGA, D., and MENARD, S. *Multiple Problem Youth.* Springer, 1989.

EMERY, R. E. Family violence. *American Psychologist* (1989) 44:321–28.

FINNEGAN, W. A street kid in the drug trade. *The New Yorker.* September 10, 1990, pp. 51–86; September 17, 1990, pp. 60–90.

FOSTER, B. *The urban school in the modern metropolis.* Presentation at the University of Hartford. October 10, 1990.

GERBNER, G., GROSS, L., SIGNIORELLI, N., and MORGAN, M. Television's mean world: Violence profile no. 14–15. (University of Pennsylvania, Annenberg School of Communication). In R. M. Liebert and J. Sprafkin, *The Early Window* 3rd ed. Pergamon, 1986.

GORDON, L. *Heroes of Their Own Lives: The Politics and History of Family Violence.* Viking, 1988.

GRAHAM, H. D., and GURR, T. R. *Violence in America: Historical and Comparative Perspectives. Report submitted to the National Commission on the Causes and Prevention of Violence.* Bantam, 1969.

HAMMER, M. C. *Please Hammer don't hurt 'em.* New York: Bust-It Publishing (BMI), 1990.

Hartford Courant. FCC study targeting TV for kids. November 9, 1990.

HEAROLD, S. A synthesis of 1043 effects of television on social behavior. In G. Comstock, ed., *Public Communication and Behavior.* Academic Press, 1986, pp. 65–133.

HUESMANN, L. R., and ERON, L. D. *Television and the Aggressive Child: A Cross-National Comparison.* Erlbaum, 1986a.

HUESMANN, L. R., and ERON, L. D. The development of aggression in American children as a consequence of television violence viewing. In L. R. Huesmann and L. D. Eron, eds., *Television and the Aggressive Child: A Cross-National Comparison.* Erlbaum, 1986b, pp. 45–80.

HUIZINGA, D. *Demographic characteristics and delinquent behavior of emotionally disturbed and violent adolescents.* Paper prepared for Conference on Emotionally Disturbed and Aggressive/Violent Adolescents, Durham, NC, 1987.

KLECK, G. Prepared testimony, Select Committee on Children, Youth and Families, U.S. House of Representatives, June 15, 1989a.

KLECK, G. Policy lessons from recent gun control research: *Law and Contemporary Problems*, 1986. In Hearing Transcript, Select Committee on Children, Youth and Families, U.S. House of Representatives, June 15, 1989b.

KUBEY, R., and CSIKSZENTMIHALYI, M. *Television and the Quality of Life: How Viewing Shapes Everyday Experience.* Erlbaum, 1990.

LEVINGER, G., et al. Media violence an antisocial behavior. *Journal of Social Issues*, Special Issue (1986) 42:1–99.

LIEBERT, R. M., and SPRAFKIN, J. *The Early Window*, 3rd ed. Pergamon, 1988.

MCGUIRE, W. J. The myth of massive media impact: savagings and salvagings. In G. Comstock, ed., *Public Communication and Behavior*, Vol 1 (pp. 173–257). Academic Press, 1986.

MCNAMARA, E. F., KURTH, T., and HANSEN, D. Smokey Bear. In R. E. Rice, and C. K. Atkin, eds., *Public Communication Campaigns.* Sage, 1989, pp. 215–17.

MEYROWITZ, J. *No Sense of Place.* Oxford, 1985.

MITGANG, L. (Associated Press). Country kids more at risk of failure than urban youths. *West County Times*, Pinole, CA, May 23, 1990.

NIGHTINGALE, E. O., and WOLVERTON, L. *Adolescent rolelessness in modern society.* Working paper, Carnegie Council on Adolescent Development. Washington, DC, 1988.

O'KEEFE, G. J., and REID, K. The McGruff Crime Prevention Campaign. In R. E. Rice and C. K. Atkin, eds., *Public Communication Campaigns.* Sage, 1989, pp. 210–12.

PALMER, E., L., and DORR, A. *Children and the Faces of Television: Teaching, Violence, Selling.* Academic Press, 1980, pp. 81, 201–17.

PEARL, D., BOUTHILET, L., and LAZAR, J. *Television and Behavior: Ten Years of Scientific Progress and Implications for the Eighties*, Vols. 1–2. National Institute of Mental Health, 1982.

POSTMAN, N. The day our children disappear: Predictions of a media ecologist. *Phi Delta Kappan.* January 1981, pp. 382–86.

REARDON, P. T. Child-spanking not as prevalent. *Hartford Courant*, April 28, 1990.

REISS, D. Psychiatry: A change in course. *Psychiatry* (1986) 49:97–103.

ROSENTHAL, R. Media violence, antisocial behavior, and the social consequences of small effects. *Journal of Social Issues* (1986) 42:141–53.

SCHORR, L. B. *Within Our Reach: Breaking the Cycle of Disadvantage.* Anchor, 1989.

SINGER, J. L., and SINGER, D. G. *Television Imagination and Aggression: A Study of Preschoolers.* Erlbaum Associates, 1981, pp. 147ff.

STRAUS, M. A general systems theory approach to a theory of violence between family members. *Social Science Information* (1973) 12:105–25.

STRAUS, M., and GELLES, R. J. *Physical Violence in American Families.* Transaction, 1990.

STRAUS, M., GELLES, R. J., and STEINMETZ, S. K. *Behind Closed Doors: Violence in the American Family.* Anchor Books, 1980.

TUAN, Y-F. *Landscapes of Fear.* Pantheon Books, 1979.

U.S. CONGRESS. H. R. 1677, Children's Television Act of 1989, 1990.

VAN DER VOORT, T. H. A. *Television Violence: A Child's-Eye View.* Elsevier, 1986.

WIDOM, C. S. The cycle of violence. *Science* (1989) 244:160–65.

ZILLMANN, D. *Hostility and Aggression.* Erlbaum, 1979.

Child Sexual Abuse: A Model of Chronic Trauma

Frank W. Putnam and Penelope K. Trickett

ALTHOUGH there is a general consensus among concerned professionals that exposure to community violence is likely to be stressful and may contribute significantly to immediate and long-term mental health problems, there is virtually no empirical research on either its acute or enduring effects. In the absence of data, investigators planning research in this area must look to other studies of the impact of chronic environmental trauma on children, including the effects of war and child maltreatment. Research on child abuse provides an important source of information on the effects of trauma on children because it draws on both prospective and retrospective studies crossing a variety of theoretical perspectives and disciplines. The existence of data on both the acute impact of abuse on children and its chronic effects and outcomes in adults informs the generation of developmentally based psychological and biological hypotheses. This paper utilizes data from research on the acute and chronic effects of sexual abuse to discuss three broad hypotheses that may be relevant to the study of the effects of community violence on children.

CHILD SEXUAL ABUSE AS A MODEL OF CHRONIC CHILDHOOD TRAUMA

Demographics and Risk Factors

Child sexual abuse (CSA), particularly incest and other familial sexual abuse, is a major source of chronic trauma for large numbers of children in the United States. Although methodological issues complicate the comparison of many studies conducted to date, there are sufficient data to conclude that CSA is a widespread problem with an incidence of at least 160,000 cases per year (National Center for Child Abuse and Neglect 1988; U.S. Advisory Board on Child Abuse and Neglect 1990). A number of retrospective studies suggest the possibility of very high prevalence rates for CSA. For example, two large-scale studies both report prevalence rates in excess of 25% (Finkelhor, Hotaling, Lewis, and Smith 1990; Russell 1986). Retrospective prevalence studies generally report much higher rates than incidence studies because they include many cases not reported to official agencies.

In addition to incidence and prevalence data, recent studies have identified risk factors and important characteristics of sexual abuse. Retrospective studies, in particular, have yielded a number of

Frank W. Putnam, MD, is Senior Investigator at the Laboratory of Developmental Psychology, National Institute of Mental Health, Bethesda, MD.

Penelope K. Trickett, PhD, is at the Department of Psychology, University of Southern California, Los Angeles, CA.

Address correspondence to: Frank W. Putnam, Bldg 15K, NIMH, 9000 Rockville Pike, Bethesda, MD 20892.

abuse-specific variables (e.g., age of onset, frequency, type of CSA, relationship with perpetrator) that are being prospectively investigated in acute and longitudinal outcome studies (Trickett and Putnam in press). Virtually every study finds that females are sexually abused about three to four times more often than males. Although sexual abuse can occur at any point from infancy through adolescence, the peak incidence in girls is prior to puberty and centers around 7 to 8 years of age, with a mean duration of about 2 years (Conte and Schuerman 1988; Finkelhor 1979; Kendall-Tackett and Simon 1988). Girls are most often abused by a family member.

For males, the typical situation is different. Boys are likely to be abused at earlier ages, for shorter durations, and the perpetrator is more often a stranger or nonrelative. For all children, poverty is an important risk factor, increasing incidence about 4- to 7-fold (Finkelhor and Baron 1986). For girls, other risk factors include: (1) the presence of a stepfather, (2) a sexually punitive mother, (3) living separately from the mother, (4) emotional distance from the mother, and (5) having two or fewer childhood friends (Finkelhor and Baron 1986).

Outcomes Associated with Child Sexual Abuse

The vast majority of researchers report significant acute and chronic negative effects in both clinical and nonclinical samples (Briere and Runtz 1988; Browne and Finkelhor 1986; Cole and Putnam 1992; Coons 1986). The diverse nature of these outcomes initially led investigators to conclude that the effects of CSA were relatively nonspecific. Recent research has demonstrated, however, that there are a number of adult psychiatric outcomes that may be directly related to CSA including: (1) borderline personality disorder (Bryer, Nelson, Miller, and Krol 1987; Gross, Doerr, Caldirola, Guzinski, and Ripley 1980–81; Herman, Perry, and van

der Kolk 1989; Stone 1990); (2) eating disorders (Coons, Bowman, Pellow, and Schneider 1989; Goldfarb 1987; Hall, Tice, Beresford, Wolley, and Hall 1989; Schechter, Schwartz, and Greenfeld 1987); (3) multiple personality disorder (Coons 1986; Putnam 1989; Ross, Norton, and Wozney 1989; Schultz, Braun, and Kluft 1989); (4) somatization disorder (Bryer et al. 1987; Gross et al. 1980–81; Loewenstein 1990; Walker, Katon, Harrop-Griffths, Holm, Russo, and Hickok 1988) and (5) substance abuse in females (Ladwig and Anderson 1989; Root 1989; Young 1990). In addition to psychiatric outcomes, victims of CSA experience numerous interpersonal problems and maladaptive behaviors that impede their productivity and quality of life (Briere and Runtz 1988; Cole and Putnam 1992).

From a categorical perspective, the outcomes associated with CSA appear to be quite divergent. One may ask, What do eating disorders, dissociative disorders, somatoform disorders, substance abuse disorders, and Axis II personality disorders have in common? Dimensionally, however, there are a number of core psychopathological features that are shared by these different diagnostic groups. Disturbances in sense of self (e.g., low self-esteem, disturbances of identity, distortion of body image, etc.) are involved in all of these disorders ranging from the identity diffusion of borderline personality disorder to the fragmentation of self central to multiple personality disorder (Cole and Putnam 1992; Putnam 1990). Profound distortions in body image can occur in the eating, dissociative, and somatoform disorders (Horne, Van Vactor, and Emerson 1991). All of these disorders exhibit high rates of self-destructive behavior including: self-mutilation, suicide attempts, and risk taking, which reflect core problems with self-esteem, internal conflicts, and estrangement from self.

Modulation of mood and regulation of behavioral state are impaired in all of the disorders associated with CSA. Rapid mood swings, episodes of binging and purging, intermittent depression, psychodynamic splitting, alter personality state switching, and dependence on illicit substances for induction of altered states of consciousness all reflect the varying forms of precipitous and unpredictable shifts in affect and behavior experienced by victims of CSA. These rapid and uncontrollable shifts in psychological state contribute in multiple ways to the fragmentation of self and behavior characteristic of child abuse victims. They also give rise to a set of compensatory behaviors that seek to damp out the violent swings in mood and behavior. Unfortunately, many of these compensatory behaviors are highly maladaptive, for example, the frequent report by CSA victims that they use self-mutilation to break the intensely dysphoric states of depersonalization that often come over them (Coons and Milstein 1990; Favazza 1987; Greenspan and Samuel 1989; Raine 1982). Pao (1969) in his seminal article coining the syndrome of delicate self-cutting, keenly observed that these behaviors typically occurred in an altered state of consciousness that differed from depersonalization in that self-awareness was often obliterated rather than heightened but detached as is characteristic of classic depersonalization.

Research on the acute impact of CSA in children is less clear-cut. On first evaluation, half or more of sexually abused children will appear asymptomatic (Tufts 1984). In symptomatic children, the most common problems are: fears, anxiety, phobias, sleep and eating disturbances, poor self-esteem, depression, self-mutilation, suicide, anger, hostility, aggression, violence, running away, truancy, delinquency, increased vulnerability to revictimization, substance abuse, teenage prostitution, and early pregnancy (Browne and Finkelhor 1986; Conte and Schuerman 1988; Coons 1986; Edwall, Hoffmann, and Harrison 1989; Frederich, Grambsch, and Koverola 1989; Harrison, Hoffman, and Edwall 1989; Singer and Petchers 1989; White, Halpin, Strom, and Santilli 1988; Wolfe, Gentile, and Wolfe 1989). The variability and diversity of re-

ported outcomes may result in part because of: (1) inadequate sampling of subjects and measures, (2) improper analyses to control for extraneous effects, (3) the heterogeneity of the nature and severity of the CSA across different studies, and (4) differences in developmental stage both for the onset and experience of CSA and for outcome evaluations across different studies (Conte and Schuerman 1988; Trickett and Putnam in press).

Similarities and Differences between Child Sexual Abuse and Community Violence

Incest is a form of CSA that shares a number of general features with community violence, though it clearly differs in important ways discussed below. CSA shares the elements of pervasiveness of threat and chronicity of stress with community violence. The chronicity of stress and the likelihood of future traumatization common to both CSA and community violence may tap similar coping mechanisms such seeking "safe" places or escape into daydreaming and fantasy. The experience of community violence may resemble CSA in that the child lives in a situation where he or she is continually socially exposed to current or potential traumatizers with attendant stress and anxiety. Evading traumatization requires continual vigilance and active escape behaviors, which must necessarily take precedence over other activities and interests. Clinical work with CSA victims indicates that safety seeking is a constant cognitive, emotional, and behavioral preoccupation for the sexually abused child. In situations where there is no possibility of physical escape, dissociation may serve as a psychological escape that detaches the child from the horror of the experience. My (F.W.P.) consultation experiences in the classrooms of inner-city Washington, DC, suggests to me that dissociation is common among children exposed to high levels of community violence (Putnam in press).

The pervasiveness of threat accompanying both sources of trauma may induce similar physiological stress reactions. CSA is generally characterized by multiple traumatic episodes and numerous social encounters with perpetrators. The mathematics of incest dictate that most children experience tens to hundreds of separate traumatic episodes. For example, in our study of sexually abused girls, starting around a mean of age 8.7 years, the average child was abused for 24.12 months with a frequency of about one episode per 3 weeks for an average of about 35 episodes (Putnam and Trickett 1987–88). The range and frequencies of traumatic episodes are not yet known for community violence but, like CSA, these statistics may not really represent the full extent of trauma. CSA survivors often describe the unceasing anxiety about possible or impending abuse as more stressful than the actual episodes. The lack of safe environments and/or separations from situations or individuals guaranteeing safety can be profoundly traumatic experiences for helpless children. Children surrounded by the constant and often unpredictable dangers of community violence are likely obsessed with analogous anxieties and concerns for safety.

CSA probably differs from community violence in the degree of family support available to the child. One would anticipate that a substantial percentage of children exposed to community violence can count on the relative safety of their home, in contrast to incest victims where the home usually represents the place of gravest danger. Family and community supports are more likely to acknowledge the dangers and intervene in community violence situations in ways not available to incest victims, who frequently dare not share their secret with anyone. Unlike community violence, disclosure of familial sexual abuse often has serious traumatic sequelae in and of itself, for example, the breakup of the family unit, placement in foster care or other separations from parents and family, intrusion of social service system into the family process, and involvement in the criminal justice system

(Sauzier 1989). The demographics of CSA likely differ from community violence in the relatively higher exposure of females to sexual abuse compared to males.

The nature of the traumatic experience differs in important ways also. CSA involves violations of physical, sexual, psychological, and social relationship boundaries. The child may be physically forced and/or emotionally coerced into active participation and may witness or even participate in the abuse of siblings. The recurrent violations of bodily boundaries, in particular, may lead to a range of disturbances in sense of self that are not shared by community violence victims (Putnam 1990). And of course, the transgressions of generational boundaries inherent in CSA and their impact on the child's working models of social relationships probably have little counterpart in community violence.

A DEVELOPMENTAL PERSPECTIVE ON THE EFFECTS OF CHILD SEXUAL ABUSE

Although knowledge of the developmental effects of childhood sexual abuse is too sparse to permit the articulation of a comprehensive theory of its effects, the current data do provide a basis for generating several sets of propositions that taken together constitute a theoretical orientation toward research on CSA and, by extension, to other forms of chronic trauma. Coarse-grained analyses of the impact of CSA on different developmental stages suggest that prepubertal abuse has more profound long-term effects than postpubertal abuse (Courtouis 1979; Finkelhor 1979; Meiselman 1978; Russell 1986; Wolfe et al. 1989), though some investigators do not find significant stage-related effects (Browne and Finkelhor 1986).

Developmental and personality research indicates that the psychological effects of CSA are likely to be manifest in a number of interrelated areas involving: (1) the development of self-esteem and self-concepts; (2) beliefs about personal power, control, and self-efficacy; (3) development of cognitive and social competencies; (4) emotional and behavioral regulation; and (5) psychiatric symptomatology. Self-image and body image are powerfully impacted by CSA (Cole and Putnam 1992; Morgan and Froning 1990; Putnam 1990). The intrinsic powerlessness associated with CSA may result in a diminishment of the child's developing sense of his or her competencies, locus of control, and efficacy (Trickett and Putnam in press). Profoundly disturbing experiences may heighten emotional reactivity, produce emotional numbness and detachment, or result in a cyclic alternation between these two extremes as is often manifest in post-traumatic stress disorder (PTSD – van der Kolk 1987).

The pubertal period in particular appears to be a critical developmental transition period around which to focus investigation as it contains a number of developmental tasks likely impacted by abuse experiences including: (1) attainment of a new and positive sense of self; (2) establishment of strong, intimate interpersonal relationships, particularly with peers, and especially with those of the opposite sex; and (3) beginning the process of developing independence from the family of origin (Simmons, Blyth, and McKinney 1983; Trickett and Putnam in press). Puberty encompasses a 3- to 4-year span characterized by profound changes in body size, appearance, and physiology coupled with the onset of powerful new hormonal factors influencing emotional and sexual responses. Even in normal, nontraumatized children this can be a stressful period notable for emotional and behavioral turmoil (Hamburg 1974; Petersen 1988; Petersen and Taylor 1980). Many of the family factors (e.g., a warm, supportive family environment) that moderate the passage through puberty in normal children, and which may well also be present for victims of community violence, are typically absent in CSA (Trickett and Putnam in press).

The pubertal period is also a time of exceedingly rapid physical growth and physiological change. Any stress-induced hormonal or biological responses produced by CSA would occur in the context of newly maturing hormonal systems; for example, the activation of the hypothalamic–pituitary–gonadal (HPG) axis is a central event in puberty (Persky 1987). The effect of chronic stress on the activation and maturation of these systems and the setting of thresholds or other parameters influencing sensitivity and reactivity to environmental events is virtually unknown in humans. Recent research on posttraumatic stress disorder (PTSD) indicates that there are long-term biological alterations produced by exposure to trauma, for example, chronic increases in heart rate (Pitman, Orr, Forgue et al. 1987; Pitman, van der Kolk, Orr et al. 1990; van der Kolk 1987). Given these physiological alterations in adults exposed to circumscribed and comprehensible experiences (e.g., an airplane crash or a night club fire), one may reasonably speculate that exposure to chronic stressors and recurrent trauma in childhood is equally likely to produce significant biological sequelae. Further research on the physiology of normal growth and development, and on the biological responses of children and adolescents to stress is crucial to our understanding of an array of potentially far-reaching biological effects of chronic trauma.

POSSIBLE MECHANISMS MEDIATING THE EFFECTS OF TRAUMA

Dissociation

Dissociation is a complex psychophysiological process manifest by a disruption in the normally integrative processes of memory, identity, and consciousness (American Psychiatric Association 1987). Dissociation is conceptualized as occurring along a continuum ranging from the normal, minor dissociations of everyday life such as momentarily spacing out or daydreaming to pathological manifestations such as the profound disruptions in self and memory that occur in multiple personality disorder or psychogenic fugue states. Evidence for the existence of a dissociative continuum comes from studies of normal and psychiatric populations with measures such as the Dissociative Experiences Scale (DES—Bernstein and Putnam 1986; Chu and Dill 1990; Ross, Miller, Bjornson, Reagor, Fraser, and Anderson 1990).

Clinical work with a variety of trauma victims including torture, combat post-traumatic stress disorder, and victims of natural disasters and child abuse indicates that the defensive use of dissociation against overwhelming trauma is common and is probably a fundamental psychological capacity (Bliss 1986; Braun and Sachs 1985; Briere and Conte 1989; Chu and Dill 1990; Coons 1986; Kluft 1985; Ludwig 1983; Putnam 1985; Ross et al. 1989; Spiegel 1991; Stern 1984). Dissociation appears to serve a number of highly protective functions in the face of intolerable pain, fear, or horror. Ludwig's enumeration of these functions includes: (1) the automatization of certain behaviors; (2) the resolution of irreconcilable conflicts; (3) escape from the constraints of reality; (4) isolation of catastrophic experiences; and (5) the cathartic discharge of certain feelings (Ludwig 1983). Individuals in dissociated states of consciousness are often analgesic for pain. The experience of profound depersonalization that accompanies a traumatically induced dissociated state of consciousness serves to psychologically distance the individual from the situation so that it is experienced "as if it were happening to someone else and I was watching from a safe place."

The relative genetic and environmental contributions to dissociative capacities has not been established. There is reason to believe that dissociation is a capacity that is strongly influenced by environmental factors and may be transmitted transgenerationally primarily by behavioral rather than genetic mechanisms, but the necessary studies have not yet been done (Morgan 1973; Putnam 1991a). There is also interest in the possibility that increased levels of dissociation in parents may increase the likelihood of their abusing their own children (Egeland, Jacobvitz, and Sroufe 1988; Putnam 1991a). And lastly, one should not discount the possibility that children and parents mutually stimulate dissociative behavior in each other, for example, the division of attention necessary to perform a complex task while monitoring the roamings of a toddler and "tuning-out" behaviors in both parents and children. Studies of normal and pathological dissociation in children are underway using the Child Dissociative Checklist (CDC) and other clinically derived measures and interviews (Putnam, Helmers, and Trickett in press).

At the present time, our understanding of pathological dissociation in traumatized children and adolescents is based on clinical experience rather than on systematic study. Recent case series of children and adolescents with dissociative disorders indicate that they share a number of common symptoms and behaviors (Bowman 1990; Dell and Eisenhower 1990; Fagan and McMahon 1984; Hornstein and Putnam in press; Hornstein and Tyson 1991; Kluft 1985; Peterson 1990; Putnam 1991a; Riley and Mead 1988; Vincent and Pickering 1988b). Spontaneous trance-like states, in which the child is inattentive and unresponsive, are probably the single most common dissociative symptom in children. These blank spells impact significantly on school work and other arenas of cognitive performance (Dell and Eisenhower 1990; Fagan and McMahon 1984; Peterson 1990; Putnam 1991a). Usually the child has no awareness of this behavior but may be cognizant of missing information that peers know. In addition to missing important information, these dissociative gaps in the continuity of experience may contribute to an impairment in cause–effect reasoning and the failure to learn from experience commonly observed in dissociating children and adults (Putnam 1989, 1991a).

Perplexing shifts in the child's fund of knowledge, skills, or abilities are widely reported by caretakers and teachers (Dell and Eisenhower 1990; Fagan and McMahon 1984; Peterson 1990; Putnam 1991a).

These often rapid shifts in mental and physical abilities appear to reflect dissociative state-dependent learning and memory retrieval processes that produce erratic retrieval of certain types of memory storage, particularly implicit (procedural) and autobiographical memory (Nissen, Ross, Willingham, Mackenzie, and Schacter 1988; Putnam, 1991b; Schacter, Kihlstrom, Kihlstrom, and Berren 1989). The child experiences erratic access to important information or abilities, which produces wide swings in performance of cognitive and manual skills. The child's subjective response is to feel "stupid," because no matter how hard these children try, they cannot seem to improve their performance: Even after exhaustive study, they are just as likely to draw a blank when taking the examination. This, of course, has major ramifications for self-esteem.

Problems with regulation of behavior and affect are common in childhood dissociative disorders (Dell and Eisenhower 1990; Fagan and McMahon 1984; Peterson 1990; Putnam 1991a; Venn 1984; Vincent and Pickering 1988a; Weiss, Sutton, and Utecht 1985). Adults with dissociative disorders likewise manifest marked mood swings, intermittent depression, panic attacks, and other precipitous shifts in affective and behavioral state (Bliss 1986; Coons, Bowman, and Milstein 1988; Putnam 1989; Ross et al. 1989; Schultz et al. 1989). The switching of the alter personalities of multiple personality disorder (MPD) patients is an extreme example of rapid shifts in psychological state that are a core feature of the dissociative disorders. These little-studied phenomena interestingly share many psychophysiological properties in common with shifts in affective state (Putnam 1988). The larger questions of regulation of affect and behavioral state involve developmental tasks that are poorly understood at present, but that are highly likely to be negatively affected by traumatic experiences (Campos, Campos, and Barrett 1989; Labouvie-Vief, Hakim-Larson, DeVoe, and Schoeberlein 1989; Sroufe 1984; Wolff 1987).

Disruption of identity, though less discernible in children with their more contextually based senses of self, is apparent in childhood dissociative disorders (Dell and Eisenhower 1990; Fagan and McMahon 1984; Peterson 1990; Putnam 1991a; Venn 1984; Vincent and Pickering 1988a; Weiss et al. 1985). Consolidation of identity is an important developmental task. Clinical experience with the affective and dissociative disorders suggests that, to some extent, subjective sense of identity is a state-dependent process. Many important components of identity (e.g., self-esteem, body image, sense of personal efficacy) change dramatically with shifts in affective or dissociative state. The swings from the grandiosity of mania to the worthlessness of depression and the disparate collection of warring selves represented by the alter personalities of MPD patients typify state-dependent aspects of identity. Trauma and stress-evoked dissociation are likely to produce disruptions in the stability of identity by: (1) producing extreme affective and dissociative states with concomitant distortions of identity, (2) interfering with the long-term regulation of affect and behavior, (3) blocking retrieval of autobiographical memories which are important for continuity of self, and (4) creation of social situations that impact negatively on self-esteem.

Dissociation, then, can be understood as a natural capacity that waxes and wanes over the course of normal development, and that may be utilized by traumatized children to escape from overwhelming experiences. Frequent or prolonged use of dissociative defenses is believed to seriously impair the consolidation of identity and continuity of memory in trauma victims. Given the ubiquity of dissociative responses in adults to many forms of trauma, it is likely that children faced with the multiple and pervasive threats associated with community violence would also exhibit increased levels of dissociative behavior. Current measures of dissociative behavior in children are sufficiently reliable and valid to warrant their inclusion in studies of the impact of community violence on children's behavior (Putnam et al. in press).

Stress and Alterations in the Hormonal Milieu

Surprisingly little is known about the normal maturation of endocrine systems with growth and development, and their possible aberrant development in the face of stress and trauma. Endocrine disorders such as psychosocial dwarfism are dramatic examples of childhood environmental stressors producing profound effects on growth and development. Recent studies have examined the relationship between environmental stressors, physiological responses to stress, and behavioral and psychiatric problems (for a review, see Susman, Nottelmann, Dorn, Inoff-Germain, and Chrousos 1989). Most of these studies have focused on the hypothalamic–pituitary–adrenal (HPA) axis and the hypothalamic–pituitary–gonadal (HPG) axis. These two major endocrine axes are interconnected and sensitive to stress.

CSA or community violence can be conceptualized as a chronically stressful experience that is likely to impact on the HPA and HPG systems. Hormonal markers of such a stress response may be similar to those reported in depression, eating disorders, and physically stressed adolescent populations (e.g., athletes and ballet dancers). This would include: elevated cortisol levels, elevated androstenedione ($\Delta 4$-AD), decreased levels of luteinizing hormone (LH), decreased testosterone levels (T), and decreased dihydroepiandrosterone (DHEA) levels (Trickett and Putnam in press). Many of these hormones (e.g., cortisol, testosterone, DHEA, and D-AD) have behavioral effects, most robustly demonstrated in males. For example, increased aggression, a consistently reported effect of physical and sexual abuse, may be related to alterations in hormonal levels. In nonclinical samples, aggressive behavior and acting out have been correlated with lower gonadal steroid and higher Δ-AD levels in boys. Susman et al. reported that acting out behaviors in

adolescents were associated with lower estradiol (E_2) levels and lower testosterone-to-estradiol ratios (T/E_2) (Susman, Inoff-Germain, Nottelmann, Cutler, Loriaux, and Chrousos 1987). Future studies should investigate these and other potential hormonal correlates as possible biological factors contributing to behavioral problems in traumatized children.

Preliminary data from our prospective, longitudinal study of sexually abused girls indicate that as a group they have significantly higher morning cortisol levels than their sex-, age-, race-, SES-, and family constellation-matched controls, and that this elevation is still present a year or more after the abuse has been disclosed to a child protective services agency (Putnam et al. 1991). Cortisol, a steroid hormone secreted by the adrenal cortex, has a range of significant behavioral, cognitive, and even genetic effects (Yehuda, Giller, Southwick, Lowy, and Mason 1991). Cortisol is implicated in cognitive deficits; alterations in the maturation of the CNS, including changes in receptor density and type; and even the activation of certain regulatory genes involved in regulation of the metabolism of neurotransmitters such as dopamine. Persistent elevations of cortisol have also been associated with neuronal loss in hippocampus and other areas of the brain associated with memory storage (Saplolsky, Krey, and McEwen 1985).

Studies of parental loss in childhood suggest that alterations in cortisol may be lifelong as a result of alterations in basic feedback threshold regulatory mechanisms (Breier, Kelsoe, Kirwin, Beller, Wolkowitz, and Pickar 1988). Robert Pynoos has suggested that the elevated cortisol levels in sexually abused girls may be secondary to loss of parental objects (i.e., the loss of their father and/or mother as a result of the incest or the social repercussions of disclosure of incest) rather than attributable to posttraumatic stress effects (Pynoos – Public comments made at the Community Violence Symposium, November 1990). Stress-induced or object loss-induced alterations of the HPA axis could conceivably produce lifelong increased vulnerability to stress and result in far-reaching perturbations in the maturation of neuroendocrine systems.

Trauma-Induced Alterations in Growth and Development

It is possible that similar stress-induced physiological disturbances may affect the timing and/or rate of physical development in traumatized children. Activation of the HPA axis has well-described effects on the HPG axis including the suppression of gonadal hormones. Stress-related effects on the HPG axis include alterations in the timing and progression of physical growth, timing of puberty (particularly menarche and regularity of menstrual cycles in females), and cognitive, social, and emotional development mediated through direct and indirect effects (Susman et al. 1989). Much of the data from animal and human studies (e.g., girls training to be ballet dancers—Brooks-Gunn and Ruble 1983) would suggest that stress activation of the HPA system would suppress or delay sexual maturation. Other studies, however, such a Surbey's large-scale questionnaire study of Canadian adolescents, have found that stress can be significantly associated with earlier menarche (Surbey 1990). Belsky, Steinberg, and Draper (1990), reviewing existing research, find evidence of a connection between stress and earlier menarche, which they suggest may have an evolutionary basis (Belsky, Steinberg, and Draper, 1990). A test of this model using data from a longitudinal study of 16-year-old girls are partially confirmatory (Moffit, Caspi, Belsky, and Silva 1992).

Among clinicians working with sexually abused girls, there is the widespread impression that these children undergo earlier physical maturation. To date, only one study has attempted to systematically investigate this possibility. Herman-Giddens and colleagues found a 1 in 15 incidence of the onset of puberty prior to age 8 in a sample of 105 sexually abused girls (Herman-Giddens, Sandler, and Friedman

1988). In all but one of these early-developing girls there was evidence of vaginal penetration. The authors speculated that the penetration associated with the sexual abuse "may be a stressor that in some way stimulates adrenal androgen secretion or early activation of the hypothalamic–pituitary axis" (p. 433). Elsewhere, Trickett and Putnam (in press) have speculated on the possibility that genital contact and penetration may expose the girls to male pheromones that have been shown to induce significantly earlier sexual maturation of females in animal studies (Vandenbergh 1969; Vandenbergh, Whitsett, and Lonbardi 1975). Recent human studies have demonstrated that male pheromones do, in fact, affect gonadal hormonal levels in females, and some have even speculated that changing social mores have resulted in increased exposure of females to male pheromones, thus producing the well-documented decline in the age of menarche over the last three centuries (Burger and Gochfeld 1985; Cutler, Preti, Krieger, Huggins, Garcia, and Lawley 1986; Russell, Switz, and Thompson 1980; Veith, Buck, Getzlaf, Van Dalfsen, and Slade 1983).

While these mechanisms remain purely speculative at this time, they do point to potentially complex and far-reaching effects of traumatization in childhood. If trauma affects growth and development—for example, results in earlier sexual maturation in sexually abused girls—then there are a host of secondary consequences resulting from nonalignment in development with peers. For example, studies of normal growth and development indicate that early developing girls have lower self-esteem, fewer girlfriends, and more older boyfriends, and are at higher risk for substance abuse and early pregnancy. All of these outcomes have, of course, already been associated with sexual abuse in girls. Future studies investigating the effects of community violence or other traumatic environments should at least include simple measures of growth and development to assess for possible stress-related effects on physical maturation.

Methodological Issues Inherent in Biological Measures

Although an argument has been made for the inclusion of biological measures in research on the effects of community violence on children, there are many serious methodological limitations associated with biological measures. Biological studies are expensive, time consuming, and require rigorous control of many variables for meaningful results. For many reasons, biological measures are best collected in inpatient or clinic settings where critical collection variables and preparation procedures are more easily controlled. The expense of biological measures often limits sample sizes; for example, our corticotrophin-releasing hormone (CRH) infusion study to determine the source (adrenal or hypothalamic dysfunction) of cortisol abnormalities in sexually abused girls costs over $2000 per subject, in addition to requiring the child's cooperation in collecting four separate 24-hour urine samples and submitting to a 3-hour procedure involving an indwelling intravenous catheter. Obviously such procedures are beyond the means and expertise of most social investigators interested in the effects of community violence.

Conversely, biologically oriented investigators seeking to study traumatized children are often woefully unaware of the necessity to control for relevant ecological variables to ensure generalizability of their sample. In addition, many biologically oriented researchers appear to misunderstand the essence of extended traumatic experiences such as incest. We are struck by how often they seem to regard the experience of incest as if it were like schizophrenia or some other disorder that was "caught" or "inherited" rather than inflicted upon a child. Perhaps the most frequent methodological suggestion made by biologically oriented researchers reviewing our longitudinal sexual abuse study is that we should use nonabused siblings as controls. In actual fact, it is very, very rare to find families with nonabused sibling "littermate-type" controls. It is unfor-tunately all too common to find that all the children in an incestuous family have suffered some form of abuse. Research on CSA or community violence that seeks to integrate biological perspectives and measures must remain grounded in the realities of the children, families, and communities being studied.

One obvious solution to this dilemma is the sharing of research samples by investigators from different disciplines. If community-based researchers were supported by biologically oriented collaborators located near the communities being studied, it would be possible for the social science researchers to select representative subsamples for more intensive biological studies. There is reason to believe that such collaborations could work. Early networking among researchers interested in community violence has already established working contacts across a range of diverse disciplines. In addition, early networking among potential funding sources, (e.g., the NIMH and private foundations) can be extended to actively promote the coordination of funding for biological and social science investigators working on shared samples. In most instances, the samples of interest to researchers of community violence are located in urban areas near major medical research institutions. New funding initiatives targeting community violence would serve to attract biological researchers now having difficulty obtaining grants in other areas. Prioritization of funding for collaborative, multidisciplinary studies would also increase interest in such projects.

DISCUSSION

The preceding discussion of postulated mechanisms being investigated with respect to psychiatric and behavioral outcomes of child sexual abuse is intended to inform and stimulate hypothesis generation in research on community violence. Although there are important differences between the experiences of community violence and child sexual abuse, it is likely that these two broad forms of trauma share many common elements with respect to chronicity of stress and pervasiveness of threat, and therefore may tap common psychological and physiological responses.

The long-term outcomes of exposure to community violence are not known as yet, but our more extensive experience with CSA would suggest that problems with identity, regulation of affect, modulation of behavioral state, and difficulties with attention, cognition, and memory are likely to be core problems. There may be multiple psychophysiological mechanisms contributing to these difficulties. For example, problems with attention, cognition, and memory can result from increased levels of dissociation, from clinical depression, or from high levels of corticosteriods. Disentangling causal sequences may be extremely difficult as some of these effects may be precursors for others; for example, high levels of dissociation may contribute directly and indirectly to depression, which has been associated with abnormalities of the HPA axis. Prior research with other mental disorders (e.g., schizophrenia) would indicate that there are not going to be simple, straightforward answers.

Even if none of the hypotheses presented here are especially relevant, research on the effects of community vio- lence can still profit from a thoughtful examination of the problems that have plagued research on the effects of CSA as it is likely that many of the same issues will resurface in early work on community violence. In particular, heterogeneity in the nature and severity of traumatic exposure and differences in developmental stage at the time of exposure are likely to be major confounding problems for pioneering researchers. Early work should attempt to carefully clarify the nature and types of traumatic stressors so that definitions and criteria can be standardized across studies and instruments can be developed to quantify levels of exposure. Based on experience with CSA, it is likely that there are critical developmental periods with respect to the acute impact of community violence and long-term outcomes. Research designs should seek to identify critical periods and to follow children for sufficient time to allow for the emergence of delayed "sleeper" effects such as are only now being identified for CSA. Perhaps our growing awareness of the many types of trauma and violence to which children in our society are exposed will stimulate the development of a more unified field of traumatology that integrates what is now a confusion of disciplines and perspectives on the major public health problem that confronts our nation's children (Donovan and McIntyre 1990).

REFERENCES

AMERICAN PSYCHIATRIC ASSOCIATION. *Diagnostic and Statistical Manual of Mental Disorders*, 3rd ed., rev. American Psychiatric Press, 1987.

BELSKY, J., STEINBERG, L., and DRAPER, P. *Childhood experience, interpersonal development, and reproductive strategy: An evolutionary theory of socialization.* Unpublished manuscript, Pennsylvania State University, 1990.

BERNSTEIN, E. M., and PUTNAM, F. W. Development, reliability and validity of a dissociation scale. *Journal of Nervous and Mental Disease* (1986) 174(12):727-35.

BLISS, E. L. *Multiple personality, allied disorders and hypnosis.* Oxford University Press, 1986.

BOWMAN, E. S. Adolescent multiple personality disorder in the nineteenth and early twentieth century. *Dissociation* (1990) 3(4):179-87.

BRAUN, B. G., and SACHS, R. G. The development of multiple personality disorder: Predisposing, precipitating, and perpetuating factors. In R. P. Kluft, ed., *Childhood Antecedents of Multiple Personality* (pp. 37-64). American Psychiatric Press, 1985.

BREIER, A., KELSOE, J. R., KIRWIN, P. D., BELLER, S. A., WOLKOWITZ, O. M., and PICKAR, D. Early parental loss and development of adult psychopathology. *Archives of General Psychiatry* (1988) 45:987-93.

BRIERE, J., and CONTE, J. *Amnesia in adults molested as children: Testing theories of repression.* Presented at the Annual meeting of the American Psychological Association, New Orleans, LA, August 1989.

BRIERE, J., and RUNTZ, M. Symptomatology associated with childhood sexual victimization in a nonclinical adult sample. *Child Abuse and Neglect* (1988) 12:51–59.

BROOKS-GUNN, B., and RUBLE, D. N. The experience of menarche from a developmental perspective. In J. Brooks-Gunn and A. C. Petersen, eds., *Girls at Puberty: Biological and Psychosocial Perspectives*. Plenum Press, 1983.

BROWNE, A., and FINKELHOR, D. Impact of child sexual abuse: A review of the literature. *Psychological Bulletin* (1986) 99(1):66–77.

BRYER, J. B., NELSON, B. A., MILLER, J. B., and KROL, P. A. Childhood sexual and physical abuse as factors in adult psychiatric illness. *American Journal of Psychiatry* (1987) 144(11):1426–30.

BURGER, J., and GOCHFELD, M. A hypothesis on the role of phermones on age of menarche. *Medical Hypotheses* (1985) 17:39–46.

CAMPOS, J. J., CAMPOS, R. G., and BARRETT, K. C. Emergent themes in the study of emotional development and emotion regulation. *Developmental Psychology* (1989) 25:394–402.

CHU, J. A., and DILL, D. L. Dissociative symptoms in relation to childhood physical and sexual abuse. *American Journal of Psychiatry* (1990) 147:887–92.

COLE, P. M., and PUTNAM, F. W. Effect of incest on self and social functioning: A developmental psychopathological perspective. *Journal of Consulting and Clinical Psychology* (1992) 60:174–84.

CONTE, J. R., and SCHUERMAN, J. R. The effects of sexual abuse on children. *Journal of Interpersonal Violence* (1988) 2:380–90.

COONS, P., BOWMAN, E., and MILSTEIN, V. Multiple personality disorder: A clinical investigation of 50 cases. *Journal of Nervous and Mental Disease* (1988) 176:519–27.

COONS, P. M. Psychiatric problems associated with child abuse: A review. In J. J. Jacobsen, ed., *Psychiatric Sequelae of Child Abuse*. C. C. Thomas, 1986.

COONS, P. M., BOWMAN, E. S., PELLOW, T. A., and SCHNEIDER, P. Post-traumatic aspects of the treatment of victims of sexual abuse and incest. *Psychological Clinics of North America* (1989) 12:325–35.

COONS, P. M., and MILSTEIN, V. Self-mutilation associated with dissociative disorders. *Dissociation* (1990) 3:81–87.

COURTOUIS, C. The incest experience and its aftermath. *Victimology* (1979) 4:337–47.

CUTLER, W. B., PRETI, G., KRIEGER, A., HUGGINS, G. R., GARCIA, C. R., and LAWLEY, H. J. Human axillary secretions influence women's menstrual cycles: The role of donor extract from men. *Hormones and Behavior* (1986) 20:463–73.

DELL, P. F., and EISENHOWER, J. W. Adolescent multiple personality disorder. *Journal of the American Academy of Childhood and Adolescent Psychiatry* (1990) 29:359–66.

DONOVAN, D. M., and MCINTYRE, D. *Healing the Hurt Child*. W. W. Norton, 1990.

EDWALL, G. E., HOFFMANN, N. G., and HARRISON, P. A. Psychological correlates of sexual abuse in adolescent girls in chemical dependency treatment. *Adolescence* (1989) 24:279–88.

EGELAND, B., JACOBVITZ, D., and SROUFE, L. A. Breaking the abuse cycle. *Childhood Development* (1988) 59:1080–88.

FAGAN, J., and MCMAHON, P. P. Incipent multiple personality in children: Four cases. *Journal of Nervous and Mental Disease* (1984) 172(1):26–36.

FAVAZZA, A. R. *Bodies under Seige: Self-Mutilation in Culture and Psychiatry*. Johns Hopkins University Press, 1987.

FINKELHOR, D. *Sexually Victimized Children*. Free Press, 1979.

FINKELHOR, D., and BARON, L. Risk factors for childhood sexual abuse: A review of the evidence. In D. Finkelhor, S. Araji, L. Baron, A. Browne, S. Doyle Peters, and G. E. Wyatt, eds., *A Sourcebook on Child Sexual Abuse*. Sage, 1986.

FINKELHOR, D., HOTALING, G., LEWIS, I. A., and SMITH, C. Sexual abuse in a national survey of adult men and women: Prevalence, characteristics, and risk factors. *Child Abuse and Neglect* (1990) 14:19–28.

FREDERICH, W. N., GRAMBSCH, P., and KOVEROLA, C. *Child sexual behavior inventory: A comparison of a normal and clinical population*. Paper presented at International Academy of Sex Research, Princeton, NJ, 1989.

GOLDFARB, L. A. Sexual abuse antecedent to anorexia nervosa, bulimia and compulsive eating: Three case reports. *International Journal of Eating Disorders* (1987) 6:665–80.

GREENSPAN, G. S., and SAMUEL, S. E. Self-cutting after rape. *American Journal of Psychiatry* (1989) 146:789–90.

GROSS, R. J., DOERR, H., CALDIROLA, D., GUZINSKI, G. M., and RIPLEY, H. S. Borderline syndrome and incest in chronic pelvic pain patients. *International Journal of Psychiatry in Medicine* (1980–81) 10(1):79–96.

HALL, R. C., TICE, L., BERESFORD, T. P., WOLLEY, B., and HALL, A. K. Sexual abuse in patients with anorexia nervosa and bulimia. *Psychosomatics* (1989) 30:73–79.

HAMBURG, B. A. Early adolescence: A specific and stressful stage of the life cycle. In G. V. Coelho, B. A. Hamburg, and J. E. Adams, eds., *Coping and Adaptation*. Basic Books, 1974.

HARRISON, P. A., HOFFMAN, N. G., and EDWALL, C. E. Differential drug use patterns among sexually abused adolescent girls in treatment for chemical dependency. *International Journal of the Addictions* (1989) 24:499–514.

HERMAN, J. L., PERRY, J. C., and VAN DER KOLK, B. A. Childhood trauma in borderline personality disorder. *American Journal of Psychiatry* (1989) 146(4):490–95.

HERMAN-GIDDENS, M. E., SANDLER, A. D., and FRIEDMAN, N. E. Sexual precocity in girls: An association with sexual abuse? *American Journal of Diseases of the Child* (1988) 142:431–33.

HORNE, R. L., VAN VACTOR, J. C., and EMERSON, S. Disturbed body image in patients with eating disorders. *American Journal of Psychiatry*, (1991) 148(2):211-15.

HORNSTEIN, N. L., and PUTNAM, F. W. Clinical phenomenology of child and adolescent dissociative disorders. *Journal of the American Academy of Childhood and Adolescent Psychiatry*, in press.

HORNSTEIN, N. L., and TYSON, S. Inpatient treatment of children with multiple personality/dissociative disorders and their families. *Psychiatric Clinics of North America* (1991) 14(3):631-48.

KENDALL-TACKETT, K. A., and SIMON, A. F. Molestation and the onset of puberty: Data from 365 adults molested as children. *Child Abuse and Neglect* (1988) 12:73-81.

KLUFT, R. P. Childhood multiple personality disorder: Predictors, clinical findings, and treatment results. In R. P. Kluft, ed. *Childhood Antecedents of Multiple Personality* (pp. 167-96). American Psychiatric Press, 1985.

LABOUVIE-VIEF, G., HAKIM-LARSON, J., DEVOE, M., and SCHOEBERLEIN, S. Emotions and self-regulation: A life span view. *Human Development* (1989) 32:279-99.

LADWIG, G. B., and ANDERSON, M. D. Substance abuse in women: Relationship between chemical dependency in women and past reports of physical and sexual abuse. *International Journal of the Addictions* (1989) 24:739-54.

LOEWENSTEIN, R. J. Somatoform disorders in victims of incest and child abuse. In R. P. Kluft, eds. *Incest-Related Syndromes of Psychopathology* (pp. 75-112). American Psychiatric Press, 1990.

LUDWIG, A. M. The psychobiological functions of dissociation. *American Journal of Clinical Hypnosis* 26:93-99.

MEISELMAN, K. *Incest.* Jossey-Bass, 1978.

MOFFIT, T. E., CASPI, A., BELSKY, J., and SILVA, P. A. Childhood experience and the onset of menarche: A test of a sociobiological model. *Child Development* (1992) 63:47-58.

MORGAN, A. The heritability of hypnotic susceptibility in twins. *Journal of Abnormal Psychology* (1973) 82:55-61.

MORGAN, E., and FRONING, M. L. Child sexual abuse sequelae and body-image surgery. *Plastic and Reconstructive Surgery* (1990) 86:475-80.

NATIONAL CENTER FOR CHILD ABUSE AND NEGLECT. *Study of National Incidence and Prevalence of Child Abuse and Neglect: 1988.* U.S. Department of Health and Human Services, 1988.

NISSEN, M. J., ROSS, J. L., WILLINGHAM, D. B., MACKENZIE, T. B., and SCHACTER, D. L. Memory and awareness in a patient with multiple personality disorder. *Brain and Cognition* (1988) 8:117-34.

PAO, P. The syndrome of delicate self-cutting. *Journal of Medical Psychology* (1969) 42:195-206.

PERSKY, H. *Psychoendrocrinology of Human Sexual Behavior.* Praeger, 1987.

PETERSEN, A. C. Adolescent development. *Annual Review of Psychology* (1988) 39:583-608.

PETERSEN, A. C., and TAYLOR, B. The biological approach to adolescence. In J. Adelson, ed., *Handbook of Adolescent Psychology* Wiley, 1980.

PETERSON, G. Diagnosis of childhood multiple personality. *Dissociation* (1990) 3:3-9.

PITMAN, R. K., ORR, S. P., FORGUE, D. F., et al. Psychophysiologic assessment of post-traumatic stress disorder imagery in Vietnam combat veterans. *Archives of General Psychiatry* (1987) 44: 970-75.

PITMAN, R. K., VAN DER KOLK, B., ORR, S. P., et al. Naloxone-reversible analgesic response to combat-related stimuli in post-traumatic stress disorder. *Archives General Psychiatry* (1990) 47:541-44.

PUTNAM, F. W. Pieces of the mind: Recognizing the psychological effects of abuse. *Justice for Children* (1985) 1:6-7.

PUTNAM, F. W. The switch process in multiple personality disorder and other state-change disorders. *Dissociation* (1988) 1(1):24-32.

PUTNAM, F. W. *Diagnosis and Treatment of Multiple Personality Disorder.* Guilford Press, 1989.

PUTNAM, F. W. Disturbances of "self" in victims of childhood sexual abuse. In R. P. Kluft, ed., *Incest-Related Syndromes of Adult Psychopathology* (pp. 113-32). American Psychiatric Press, 1990.

PUTNAM, F. W. Dissociative disorders in children and adolescents: A developmental perspective. *Psychiatric Clinics of North America* (1991a) 14(3): 519-32.

PUTNAM, F. W. Recent research on multiple personality disorder. *Psychiatric Clinics of North America* (1991b) 14:489-502.

PUTNAM, F. W. Dissociation in the inner city. In C. G. Fine and R. P. Kluft, eds., *Clinical Perspectives on Multiple Personality Disorder.* American Psychiatric Press, in press.

PUTNAM, F. W., HELMERS, K., and TRICKETT, P. K. Development, reliability and validity of a child dissociation scale. *Child Abuse and Neglect*, in press.

PUTNAM, F. W., and TRICKETT, P. K. The psychobiological effects of sexual abuse. In NIMH, ed., *Annual Report* (vol. 1), U.S. Department of Health and Human Services, 1987-88.

PUTNAM, F. W., TRICKETT, P. K., HELMERS, K., SUSMAN, E., DORN, L., and EVERETT, B. Cortisol abnormalities in sexually abused girls. In *New Research Abstracts*, Annual Meeting of the American Psychiatric Association, New Orleans, May 1991.

RAINE, W. J. B. Self mutilation. *Journal of Adolescence* (1982) 5:1-13.

RILEY, R. L., and MEAD, J. The development of symptoms of multiple personality disorder in a child of three. *Dissociation* (1988) 1(3):41-46.

ROOT, M. P. P. Treatment failures: The role of sexual victimizations in women's addictive behavior. *American Journal of Orthopsychiatry* (1989) 59: 542-49.

ROSS, C. A., MILLER, S. D. J., BJORNSON, L., REAGOR, P., FRASER, G., and ANDERSON, G. Structured interview data on 102 cases of multiple personality disorder from four centers. *American Journal of Psychiatry* (1990) 147:596-601.

ROSS, C. A., NORTON, G. R., and WOZNEY, K. Multiple personality disorder: An analysis of 236 cases. *Canadian Journal of Psychiatry* (1989) 84:413-18.

RUSSELL, D. E. H. *The Secret Trauma: Incest in the Lives of Girls and Women.* Basic Books, 1986.

RUSSELL, M. J. SWITZ, F. M., and THOMPSON, K. Olfactory influences on the human menstrual cycle. *Pharmacy, Biochemistry, and Behavior* (1980) 13: 737–38.

SAPLOLSKY, R. M., KREY, L. C., and McEWEN, B. S. Prolonged glucocorticoid exposure reduces hippocampal neuron number. *Journal of Neuroscience* (1985) 5:1221–26.

SAUZIER, M. Disclosure of child sexual abuse: For better or for worse. *Psychiatric Clinics of North America* (1989) 12(2):455–69.

SCHACTER, D. L., KIHLSTROM, J. F., KIHLSTROM, L. C., and BERREN, M. B. Autobiographical memory in a case of multiple personality disorder. *Journal of Abnormal Psychology* (1989) 98(4):1–7.

SCHECHTER, J. O., SCHWARTZ, H. P., and GREENFELD, D. G. Sexual assault and anorexia nervosa. *International Journal of Eating Disorders* (1987) 5: 313–16.

SCHULTZ, R., BRAUN, B. H., and KLUFT, R. P. Multiple personality disorder: Phenomenology of selected variables in comparison to major depression. *Dissociation* (1989) 2:45–51.

SIMMONS, R. G., BLYTH, D. A., and McKINNEY, K. L. The social and psychological effects of puberty on white females. In J. Brooks-Gunn and A. C. Petersen, eds., *Girls at Puberty: Biological and Psychosocial Perspectives*. Plenum Press, 1983.

SINGER, M. I., and PETCHERS, M. K. The relationship between sexual abuse and substance abuse among psychiatrically hospitalized adolescents. *Child Abuse and Neglect* (1989) 13:319–25.

SPIEGEL, D. Posttraumatic dissociative disorders. In A. Tasman, ed., *American Psychiatric Press Review of Psychiatry*. American Psychiatric Press, 1991.

SROUFE, L. A. The organization of emotional development. In K. R. Scherer and P. Ekman, eds., *Approaches to Emotion* (pp. 109–127). Erlbaum, 1984.

STERN, C. R. The etiology of multiple personality. *Psychiatric Clinics of North America* (1984) 7:149–60.

STONE, M. H. Incest in the borderline patient. In R. P. Kluft, eds. *Incest-Related Syndromes in Adult Psychopathology* (pp. 183–204). American Psychiatric Press, 1990.

SURBEY, M. K. Family composition, stress and human menarche. In F. B. Bercovitch and T. R. Zeigler, eds., *The Socioendocrinology of Primate Reproduction*. Alan R. Liss, 1990.

SUSMAN, E. J., INOFF-GERMAIN, G. E., NOTTELMANN, E. D., CUTLER, G. B., LORIAUX, D. L. and CHROUSOS, F. P. Hormones, emotional dispositions, and aggressive attributes in young adolescents. *Child Development* (1987) 58:1114–34.

SUSMAN, E. J., NOTTELMANN, E. D., DORN, L. D., INOFF-GERMAIN, G. E., and CHROUSOS, G. P. Physiological and behavioral reactivity to stress in adolescents. In G. P. Chrousos, D. L. Loriaux, and P. W. Gold, eds., *Mechanisms of Physical and Emotional Stress* (pp. 341–52). Plenum, 1989.

TRICKETT, P., and PUTNAM, F. W. The impact of child sexual abuse on females: Toward a developmental, psychobiological integration. *Psychological Science*, in press.

TUFTS DEPARTMENT OF CHILD PSYCHIATRY. *Sexually Exploited Children: Service and Research Project*. U.S. Department of Justice, 1984.

U.S. ADVISORY BOARD ON CHILD ABUSE AND NEGLECT. *Child Abuse and Neglect: Critical First Steps in Response to a National Emergency*. Department of Health and Human Services, 1990.

VAN DER KOLK, B. A., ed. *Psychological Trauma*. American Psychiatric Press, 1987.

VANDENBERGH, J. G. Effect of the presence of a male on the sexual maturation of female mice. *Endocrinology* (1969) 81:345–56.

VANDENBERGH, J. G., WHITSETT, J. M., and LONBARDI, J. R. Partial isolation of a pheromone accelerating puberty in female mice. *Journal of Reproduction and Fertility* (1975) 43:515–23.

VEITH, J. L., BUCK, M., GETZLAF, S., VAN DALFSEN, P., and SLADE, S. Exposure to men influences the occurrence of ovulation in women. *Physiology and Behavior* (1983) 31:313–15.

VENN, J. Family etiology and remission in a case of psychogenic fugue. *Family Process* (1984) 23:429–35.

VINCENT, M., and PICKERING, M. R. Multiple personality disorder in childhood. *Canadian Journal of Psychiatry* (1988a) 33:524–29.

VINCENT, M., and PICKERING, M. R. Multiple personality disorder in childhood. *Canadian Journal of Psychiatry* (1988b) 33:524–29.

WALKER, E., KATON, W., HARROP-GRIFFTHS, J., HOLM, L., RUSSO, J., and HICKOK, L. R. Relationship of chronic pelvic pain to psychiatric diagnoses and childhood sexual abuse. *American Journal of Psychiatry* (1988) 145(1):75–80.

WEISS, M., SUTTON, P. J., and UTECHT, A. J. Multiple personality in a 10-year-old girl. *Journal of the American Academy of Child and Adolescent Psychiatry* (1985) 24(4):495–501.

WHITE, S., HALPIN, B. M., STROM, G. A., and SANTILLI, G. Behavioral comparisons of young sexually abused, neglected and nonreferred children. *Journal of Clinical Child Psychology* (1988) 17:53–61.

WOLFE, V. V., GENTILE, C., and WOLFE, D. A. The impact of sexual abuse on children: A PTSD formulation. *Behavior Therapy* (1989) 20:215–28.

WOLFF, P. H. *The Development of Behavioral States and the Expression of Emotions in Early Infancy*. University of Chicago Press, (1987).

YEHUDA, R., GILLER, E. L., SOUTHWICK, S. M., LOWY, M. T., and MASON, J. W. Hypothalamic-pituitary dysfunction in posttraumatic stress disorder. *Biological Psychiatry* (1991) 30:1–18.

YOUNG, E. B. The role of incest in relapse. *Journal of Psychoactive Drugs* (1990) 22:249–58.

Toward an Ecological/Transactional Model of Community Violence and Child Maltreatment: Consequences for Children's Development

Dante Cicchetti and Michael Lynch

IN RECENT decades it has become increasingly apparent that violence affects a significant proportion of families in the United States (Bureau of Justice Statistics 1983). Violence, in fact, is becoming a defining characteristic of American society. A recent comparison of the rates of homicide among 21 developed nations indicates that the United States has the highest homicide rate in the world, and its rate is more than four times higher than the next highest rate (Fingerhut and Kleinman 1990). What is even more alarming is the high incidence of violent death and injury for children and adolescents in the United States. Acts of violence are the cause of death for over 2000 children between the ages of 0 and 19 years each year, and more than 1.5 million children and adolescents are abused by their adult caretakers each year (Christoffel 1990).

These statistics on the occurrence of violence in our society suggest that community violence is becoming a more common feature of the environment in which children are growing up. It is critical then that researchers in child development apply themselves to the question of how community violence effects children's development. Currently, little is known about the direct and indirect effects of community violence. Some of the pioneering work in this area has focused on the appearance of posttraumatic stress symptoms in children following exposure to incidences of extreme violence (Pynoos, Frederick, Nader, Arroyo, Steinberg, Eth, Nunez, and Fairbands 1987; see also Schwarz and Kowalski 1991), and on developing an epidemiology of children's exposure to community violence (Richters and Martinez this issue).

One well-established area of research that may be able to shed light on the effects of community violence is the field of studies on the consequences of child maltreatment (Cicchetti and Carlson 1989). Clearly, the study of child maltreatment is not reducible to the study of violence. It has long been recognized that child maltreatment is highly correlated with poverty environments (Garbarino and Sherman 1980; Pelton 1988). In addition, child

Dante Cicchetti is at the Mt. Hope Family Center, Department of Psychology, University of Rochester. *Michael Lynch* is at the Mt. Hope Family Center, Department of Psychology, University of Rochester. *Address reprint requests to*: Dante Cicchetti, Mt. Hope Family Center, 187 Edinburgh Street, Rochester, NY 14608.

We wish to acknowledge the Kenworthy Swift Foundation, the Spencer Foundation, and the Spunk Fund, Inc., for their generous support of our work. We also want to thank Diane Larter, Katherine Sosin, and the Monroe County Department of Social Services for their ongoing commitment to improving the quality of life for maltreating families. Finally, we want to thank Sheree Toth for her helpful suggestions and Donna Bowman for typing this manuscript.

maltreatment itself is a complex and heterogeneous phenomenon that includes both violent and nonviolent acts (Cicchetti and Barnett 1991b). Physical abuse obviously is an example of violence directed at children. Sexual abuse also may include strong elements of violence as well. However, other subtypes of child maltreatment cannot be conceptualized as violent. Physical and emotional neglect are examples of forms of maltreatment that are not characterized by violence perpetrated against children. On the other hand, many of the subtypes of child maltreatment are often comorbid (Cicchetti and Barnett 1991b).

While child maltreatment cannot be equated with violence, the study of maltreatment, its etiology, and its consequences suggests to us a model that can serve as a heuristic for investigating the effects of community violence. Such a model will allow researchers to examine how community violence and child maltreatment, either alone or in interaction, affect children's development and adaptation. The model of community violence and child maltreatment that we present has been strongly influenced by two different theoretical accounts of child maltreatment.

Cicchetti and Rizley (1981) developed a model to address the causes, consequences, and mechanisms through which maltreatment is propagated. Their model advocates a transactional approach to conceptualizing the developmental process. In a transactional model, environmental forces, caregiver characteristics, and child characteristics all influence each other and make reciprocal contributions to the events and outcomes of child development (Sameroff and Chandler 1975). Cicchetti and Rizley's model focuses on the transactions among risk factors for the occurrence of maltreatment. These risk factors are divided into two broad categories: *potentiating factors*, which increase the probability of maltreatment; and *compensatory factors*, which decrease the risk for maltreatment. Furthermore,

temporal distinctions are made for both categories of risk factors. For example, there are *transient* risk factors that fluctuate and may indicate a temporary "state." Conversely, there also are *enduring* factors that represent more permanent conditions or characteristics. According to this transactional model, maltreatment occurs only when potentiating factors outweigh compensatory ones. A more detailed description of the different type of risk factors involved in maltreatment follows.

Enduring vulnerability factors include all relatively long-lasting factors, conditions, or attributes that serve to potentiate maltreatment. These may involve parental, child, or environmental characteristics. Vulnerability factors may be biological in nature, historical (e.g., a parent with a history of being maltreated), psychological, and sociological.

Transient challengers include short-term conditions and stresses such as loss (of status, a job, or a loved one), physical injury or illness, legal difficulties, marital or family problems, discipline problems with children, and the emergence of a child into a new and more difficult developmental period.

Enduring protective factors include relatively permanent conditions that decrease the risk of maltreatment. Examples of likely protective factors include a parent's history of good parenting and a secure quality of intimate relationships between the parent figures.

Transient buffers include factors that may protect a family from stress, such as sudden improvement in financial conditions, periods of marital harmony, and a child's transition out of a difficult developmental period.

At about the same time, Belsky (1980) proposed an *ecological model* to account for the etiology of child maltreatment. This model provides a framework for defining and understanding the "ecology" or broader environment in which child maltreatment occurs. Belsky views child maltreatment as a social–psychological phenomenon that is influenced by forces within the individual, the family, the community, and the culture in which family and individual are embedded. His ecological model contains four levels of analysis: (1) ontogenic development, which includes factors within the individual that are associated with being a perpetrator of child maltreatment; (2) the microsystem, which includes factors within the family that contribute to the occurrence of child maltreatment; (3) the exosystem, which includes aspects of the communities in which families and individuals live that contribute to child maltreatment; and (4) the macrosystem, which includes the beliefs and values of the culture that contribute to the perpetuation of child maltreatment. This model has been helpful in defining the broad range of influences on the etiology of child maltreatment.

Drawing upon the Cicchetti and Rizley (1981) and the Belsky (1980) models, we present a broad and integrative explanatory framework for conceptualizing and examining the processes associated with community violence and child maltreatment, and their implications for children's development. Whereas the models that have been outlined to this point focus primarily on the *etiology* of child maltreatment, our focus is on the *outcomes* of community violence and child maltreatment and their developmental pathways. As a result, we have modified these theoretical models in accord with our emphasis on processes and sequelae. Additionally, because much of the empirical work on the effects of violence has been derived from maltreating families, our theorizing emanates largely from this base. In recognition of the combination of objective and subjective criteria used to define maltreatment phenomena, our operational definition of child maltreatment is conceptualized as treatment of children that is judged to be inappropriate and jeopardizes their growth and development (Garbarino, Guttmann, and Seeley 1986). Both potentiating and compensatory risk factors are present at each level of the ecological/transactional model. These risk factors influence the occurrence of violence in other levels of the model, as well as children's ongoing adaptation. What follows is an elaboration of our proposed model.

TOWARD AN ECOLOGICAL/TRANSACTIONAL MODEL OF COMMUNITY VIOLENCE AND CHILD MALTREATMENT

Taking an ecological/transactional perspective, we begin to see how community violence and child maltreatment interact in producing adverse consequences for children's development. Informed by both transactional and ecological models of development, we are proposing a model in which multiple levels of children's ecologies influence each other, and in turn influence children's development. In particular, with respect to the effects of violence, attitudes toward and the prevalence of violence within cultures, local communities, and families impact children's ongoing development and adaptation. The confluence of effects from culture, community, family, and previous development come together to influence developmental outcomes in children. Moreover, potentiating and compensatory risk factors associated with violence are present at each level of the ecology. These factors first determine whether violence will be present at a given level of the model. In addition, factors within a given level can influence outcomes in surrounding levels of the model. At higher, more distal levels of the ecology such as the macrosystem and the exosystem, potentiating factors increase the likelihood of community violence, whereas compensatory factors decrease the prevalence of community violence. What happens in these environmental systems also influences what occurs in the microsystem. At the level of the microsystem, potentiating and compensatory factors determine the presence or absence of violence within the family environment. Characteristics of the proximal environment have the most direct effects on children's development.

The manner in which children handle

the challenges presented by familial and community violence is seen in their own ontogenic development, which shapes their ultimate adaptation or maladaptation. An increased presence of enduring vulnerability factors and transient challengers associated with different forms of violence at all ecological levels make the successful resolution of stage salient developmental issues more problematic for children (Cicchetti, 1989). The result is an increased likelihood of negative developmental outcomes and psychopathology (Cicchetti, 1990a,b). Conversely, such an ecological/transactional model of violence and its effects also should help to account for resilient outcomes in some children. The presence of enduring protective factors and transient buffers at any level of the ecology may help to explain why some children display successful adaptation in the face of violence either within their communities or within families. Research guided by our integrative perspective can demonstrate how relevant macro- and exosystem variables impact the more proximal, microsystemic environments that mediate the influences of more distal ecological systems and have their own direct influences on children's ontogeny and ultimate adaptation.

The Macrosystem

The macrosystem subsumes cultural values and beliefs that foster violence within families and communities. Compared with other Western nations, the level of violence observed in the United States is high (Christoffel 1990; Fingerhut and Kleinman 1990; Gil 1970; Zigler 1976). In fact, violent crime continues to soar year after year (Rodino 1985). In recent years, the consensus report is that violent crime has gone up dramatically in the United States. Justice Department statistics suggest that approximately 1 out of every 10 American households is affected by violent crimes such as robbery, assault, rape, and burglary. Content analyses of films and television programs document the frequent display of violence in the United States (see Belsky 1980), supporting Straus's (1974) and Zigler's (1976, 1980) claims that violence is approved of in this country. In addition, of particular relevance for child maltreatment, physical punishment is widely practiced and condoned as a method for controlling children's behavior. As one might expect, high rates of intrafamilial violence have been identified in epidemiological surveys (Straus and Gelles, 1986). Basic to our ecological/transactional model of community violence and maltreatment is the assumption that societal willingness to tolerate such high levels of violence acts as an enduring vulnerability factor that sets the stage for the occurrence of violence in the exosystem (e.g., community violence) and microsystem (e.g., child maltreatment).

The Exosystem

The exosystem represents formal and informal social structures that impact the child's immediate environment (i.e., the microsystem) and influence what goes on in that environment (Belsky 1980). The "social structures" of the exosystem include the neighborhood, informal social networks and formal support groups, the availability of services, the availability of employment, and pervasive socioeconomic status (SES). This conceptualization of the exosystem also includes elements of Bronfenbrenner's *mesosystem*, which is comprised of the interconnections among settings such as school, peer group, church, and workplace (Bronfenbrenner 1977).

Factors within the exosystem are linked to the effects of violence in different ways. It is likely that the chronic stress and danger associated with increased community violence has serious implications for children's views of the world, themselves, and others, as well as for their moral development (Garbarino et al. 1991). However, little systematic research on the effects of pervasive violence within communities has been conducted to date. The current work of Richters and Martinez at the National Institute of Mental Health is exemplary in its attempts to delineate the links between exposure to community violence and outcomes in children. Richters and Martinez (this issue) have surveyed children and their mothers living in a violent Washington, DC, neighborhood. While a significant number of children have experienced acts of violence within their community, they are between two and four times more likely to have witnessed community violence than to have been victimized by it directly (Richters and Martinez this issue). The type of violent acts these children witnessed range from drug deals and muggings to stabbings, shootings, and murders. Furthermore, violence exposure was significantly related to distress symptoms in children such as depression and anxiety. Interestingly, the effects of exposure to violence appear to have been mediated by maternal education, with violence exposure being more strongly related to distress symptoms in children of less-educated mothers. Maternal education most likely has an organizing influence on the family environment (i.e., microsystem) and can act in either of two ways: as a potentiating factor for poor adaptation in children by not providing adequate protection against the effects of exposure to community violence, or as a compensatory factor.

In addition to having direct connections to community violence, aspects of the exosystem have implications for violence occurring within families. Sociological investigations of the etiology of child maltreatment indicate that at least two exosystem factors have significant influences on the family microsystem: the world of work and the neighborhood (Belsky 1980). Unemployment and the stress that accompany it frequently distinguish maltreating families from nonmaltreating families (Gil 1970; Parke and Collmer 1975). In fact, the majority of chronically maltreating families are found within the lowest echelons of socioeconomic status (Pelton 1978), although maltreatment is not a phenomenon solely of low SES. Economic, sociocultural, and interpersonal factors combine in these families to create

a situation of economic stress, hardship, and dependency that threatens adequate family functioning (Garbarino and Gilliam 1980; Gil 1970). In fact, a number of studies are emerging that demonstrate independent additive and interactive effects of low SES and maltreatment on children's development (Aber, Allen, Carlson, and Cicchetti 1989; Kaufman and Cicchetti 1989; Trickett, Aber, Carlson, and Cicchetti 1991; Vondra, Barnett, and Cicchetti 1990). It appears that low SES has its own independent negative effects as well as interactive effects with maltreatment that place low-SES maltreated children at risk for poor developmental outcomes. In this scenario, we see the exosystem, the microsystem, and prior ontogenic development all coming together to influence the children's adaptation.

Social isolation from neighborhood networks, support groups, and extended family also is associated with maltreatment (Garbarino 1977, 1982; Hunter and Kilstrom 1979; Kempe 1973; Parke and Collmer 1975). As a result, Kempe (1973) pointed out that maltreating families lack a "lifeline" to emotional and material support during times of stress. Also, as Garbarino and Gilliam (1980), Belsky (1984), and Sigel (1986) have pointed out, parental child-rearing practices can be influenced by information from educational institutions, the media, and social networks. If maltreating parents are isolated from the wider community, they will not be exposed to new information that could improve their child-rearing beliefs and practices (Trickett and Sussman 1988).

In discussing the association between social isolation and maltreatment, it is necessary to distinguish between the lack of support and the failure to use available support (Garbarino 1977). Several studies have indicated that the failure to use social supports is common among maltreating families (Garbarino 1977). The possible causes of social isolation involve an interaction between individual families and the environment. Relevant factors include the developmental histories of the parents, stresses that cut families off from supports, increased mobility that disrupts social networks, characteristics of the family that alienate others, the ability of neighborhoods to provide feedback and resources, and the ability of social service systems to identify and monitor high-risk families (Crittenden 1985; Crittenden and Ainsworth 1989; Garbarino 1977). In addition, based on survey data, Garbarino and Sherman (1980) found that in communities where there was a lower than expected rate of maltreatment, families experienced greater satisfaction with their neighborhoods as a context for child and family development than families from neighborhoods where maltreatment was greater than predicted. In general, parents who report dissatisfaction with the support provided by friends and neighbors likewise tend to be dissatisfied with their roles as caregivers, to engage in less optimal interactions with their children, and to provide poor-quality home environments (Corse, Schmid, and Trickett 1990; Vondra 1990). Whatever the causes of social isolation, the end result is that maltreating families are likely to be alienated from the type of support and resources that can ameliorate their family functioning. In fact, these additional supports may be especially important in the midst of the many ecological risk factors associated with poverty and low-SES membership that maltreating families face.

While studies examining the causal connections between community violence and child maltreatment are extremely difficult to conduct, several potentiating factors within the community and family can be proposed that link violence and maltreatment. Clearly a community in which violence is prevalent may contribute to the proliferation of spousal violence and child maltreatment in the family. For example, poverty and unemployment, which are often concentrated in inner-city neighborhoods, can produce increased stress and frustration that lead to violence at the broader community level and violence at the narrower family level. The finding that maltreating parents are often unemployed may also force them to live in low-income neighborhoods where the pattern of poverty, stress, and violence is focused. A question to be addressed, then, is to what extent do violent communities and maltreating families find each other? It is possible that the same type of psychological factors within parents that are associated with maltreatment draw families to communities where there is extensive violence. One specific example might be drug addiction and the violence associated with drug dealing. Drug-addicted maltreating parents may choose to live in neighborhoods where drugs are readily available, thus exposing their families to the potential of increased violence. Of course, there are many other factors that could play a role in maltreating families living in violent communities. With limited financial resources due to unemployment and low income, maltreating families may have few real opportunities to move out of violent neighborhoods. Moreover, a lack of education in many maltreating parents may further hinder their ability to gain the financial means to leave violent communities. Clearly, detailed research still is needed to delineate the associations between community violence and maltreatment.

An important point to consider in evaluating the influences of the exosystem on the maltreating family microsystem is that these potentiating factors most likely stimulate maltreatment and family dysfunction through the pressure and stress they place on families, whether the exosystem factor is a transient challenger, such as social isolation and unemployment, or is an enduring vulnerability factor such as background community violence (Belsky 1980; Garbarino 1977). To the extent that stress within the family is already high, the presence of any of these negative exosystem factors may increase the likelihood of child maltreatment. Also, if a parent's developmental history, another enduring vulnerability factor, predisposes him or her to respond to stress with aggression, then the probability of child maltreatment increases even further.

The Microsystem

Following Belsky's (1980) usage, the microsystem represents the family environment. This is the immediate context in which child maltreatment takes place (Belsky 1980). The microsystem incorporates many components, including the maltreatment itself, family dynamics, and parenting styles, as well as the developmental histories and psychological resources of the maltreating parents. However, Bronfenbrenner (1977) does not limit the microsystem to the family. According to him it includes any environmental setting that contains the developing person such as the home, school, or workplace. With this expanded conceptualization of the microsystem, forms of violence in addition to child maltreatment can be examined. In fact, according to Bronfenbrenner any violence directly experienced by children occurs within the microsystem. Theoretically, this point is significant because it places all actual experiences of violence in an ecological level that is proximal to children's ontogenic development and adaptation, suggesting that any experience of violence should have direct effects on an individual. Research on the posttraumatic stress experienced by children is relevant in this regard. Studies have documented that children exhibit posttraumatic symptoms over prolonged periods of time in response to being victimized by acts of tremendous personal violence such as being kidnapped (Terr 1981) and being on a school playground during a fatal sniper attack (Pynoos et al. 1987).

Most of our knowledge, though, on the causes and consequences of violence within the microsystem involves research on child maltreatment (Cicchetti and Howes 1991). There are a number of well-substantiated findings that indicate that the microsystems in which maltreated children develop are characterized by stressful, chaotic, and uncontrollable events.

Parents' prior developmental histories may be the first contributors to eventual family microsystems. There is considerable support for the claim that maltreating parents are more likely than nonmaltreating parents to have had a history of abuse (Conger, Burgess, and Barrett 1979; Egelan, Jacobvitz, and Paptola 1987; Hunter and Kilstrom 1979; Kaufman and Zigler 1989). It is believed that one way in which abusive parenting behaviors may be transmitted across generations is through socialization and social learning (Feshbach 1974; Hertzberger 1983). In contrast, attachment theorists claim that representational models of attachment relationships are internalized and integrated into self-structures (Bowlby 1980; Sroufe 1989; Sroufe and Fleeson 1986). As a result, these representational models may be the mechanisms through which abusive parenting is transmitted from one generation to the next. In this regard, Main and Goldwyn (1984) have found that women who remember their mothers as being rejecting are more likely to reject their own children.

The psychological resources that maltreating parents bring with them to the family ecology also distinguish them from nonmaltreating parents. Brunquell, Crichton, and Egeland (1981), in a prospective study, showed that parents who later became abusive were less psychologically complex and personally integrated than mothers who did not maltreat their children. Specifically, these mothers received less optimal scores than nonmaltreating mothers on summary scales of anxiety, locus of control, aggression, and defendence. In general, maltreating parents have been found to be depressed (Gilbreath and Cicchetti 1990; Lahey, Conger, Atkeson, and Treiber 1984), socially isolated and lacking social supports (Egeland and Brunquell 1979; Garbarino 1976, 1982; Kotelchuck 1982), and lacking in impulse control, especially when aroused and stressed (Altemier, O'Connor, Vietze, Sandler, and Sherrod 1982; Brunquell et al. 1981). Wolfe (1985) interprets these symptoms as indices of failure in psychological functioning in handling stressful life events.

Conflict may be a particularly salient feature of abusive family functioning.

Crittenden (1985) suggests that social isolation may be more characteristic in neglecting parents, whereas social conflict may be more characteristic in abusive parents. In a related vein, Trickett and Sussman (1988) found that maltreating parents report more anger and conflict in the family than nonmaltreating families. In addition, Straus, Gelles, and Steinmetz (1980) and Rosenbaum and O'Leary (1981) have observed an association between spousal violence and child maltreatment. It appears that maltreated children may witness substantial family violence as well as experience violence directed toward them (Rosenberg 1987). In general, family interactions in maltreating families are less than supportive (see Cicchetti and Howes 1991 for a review). Maltreating parents interact less with their children and display more negativity to them than do comparison parents (Burgess and Conger, 1978).

The actual parenting styles and attitudes that maltreating parents contribute to the family microsystem may have the most direct impact on children's ontogenic development. Trickett and her colleagues (Trickett, Aber, Carlson, and Cicchetti 1991; Trickett and Kuczynski 1986; Trickett and Sussman 1988) have found that maltreating parents, compared to nonmaltreating parents, are less satisfied with their children, perceive child rearing as more difficult and less enjoyable, use more controlling disciplinary techniques, do not encourage the development of autonomy in their children even though they maintain high standards of achievement, and promote an isolated life-style for themselves and their children. It is also common for maltreating parents to parentify their children, placing upon them the inappropriate expectation that the child should act as a caretaker for the parent. One of the most common characteristics of maltreated children is that they seem to have traded roles with their caregiver (Dean, Malik, Richards, and Stringer, 1986). In such parent–child relationships the child appears to be the more nurturing and sensitive member of the dyad.

In general, maltreating parents do little to foster the successful adaptation of their children on the major tasks of individual development (e.g., the formation of a secure attachment, the development of an autonomous self, the development of effective interpersonal relations, etc. – see Cicchetti 1989, 1990a, 1990b). Moreover, maltreating families do not successfully resolve the salient issues of family development (e.g., attachment, emotion regulation, autonomy, peer and school/work competence – see Cicchetti and Howes 1991 for a review). All of these negative potentiating inputs from the family microsystem may be internalized and carried forward by maltreated children as enduring vulnerability factors while they proceed through the tasks of development. Sroufe argues that whole relationships (including complex family relationships) are internalized and carried forward by the individual (Sroufe 1989; Sroufe and Fleeson 1988). As a result, it is the individual's internalized relationship history that molds one's attitudes, affects, and cognitions, thus organizing the self and shaping individual development.

Ontogenic Development

Most of the existing research relevant to an ecological/transactional model of community violence and child maltreatment has focused on the ontogenic level of the model, that is, factors within the individual that influence the achievement of competence and adaptation. At the ontogenic level, the most critical determinant of eventual competence or incompetence is the negotiation of the central issues of each developmental period (Cicchetti 1989). The manner in which these issues are handled plays a critical role in determining subsequent adaptation. Poor resolution of these issues ultimately may contribute to the development of psychopathology.

One issue of ontogenic development about which much is known regarding the effects of maltreatment is attachment (Cicchetti 1990b). The formation of a secure attachment relationship with the primary caregiver is one of the first developmental tasks that children must undertake (Ainsworth, Blehar, Waters, and Wall 1978; Bowlby 1969/1982). From an evolutionary perspective, attachment relationships serve a survival function for the initially helpless infant. Behaviors from the child's attachment system, such as crying and proximity seeking, elicit maternal response and protection. As the child becomes decreasingly helpless with the emergence of behavioral and representational abilities, the nature of the attachment relationship changes from a relationship characterized by physical proximity to one described as a "goal-corrected partnership" (Bowlby 1969/1982) where the mother and child share internal states and goals (Cicchetti, Cummings, Greenberg, and Marvin 1990). While there is ample evidence that maltreated children do form attachments, the main issues with which we are concerned are the quality of their attachments and the nature of their internal representational models of self and self in relation to others. Children form representational models of attachment figures, of themselves, and of themselves in relation to others based on their relationship history with their primary caregiver (Bowlby 1969/1982). Through these models, children's affects, cognitions, and expectations about future interactions are organized and carried forward into subsequent relationships.

Several studies have demonstrated that maltreated children form attachments to their caregivers that are more likely to be insecure than those of nonmaltreated children (Crittenden 1988; Egeland and Sroufe 1981; Schneider-Rosen, Braunwald, Carlson and Cicchetti 1985). However, a number of investigators observed patterns of behavior in the assessment of maltreated children's attachments using the Strange Situation, a standardized series of infant–mother separations and reunions covering eight 3-minute episodes (Ainsworth et al. 1978) that did not fit smoothly into the traditional A-B-C classification scheme. Crittenden (1988) noticed that a number of maltreated children in her sample who had experienced both abuse and neglect

were displaying unusual patterns of moderate-to-high levels of avoidance of the mother in combination with moderate-to-high levels of resistance. She developed a new attachment classification for these children which she labeled "A-C" avoidant/resistant, and was able to demonstrate its reliability on a separate sample of children. Main and Solomon (1986, 1990) also noticed some unusual patterns of attachment behavior in their observations of samples of maltreated children from laboratories around the country. They found a combination of moderate-to-high proximity seeking, moderate-to-high avoidance, and moderate-to-high resistance in many of their maltreated children. Unlike the case for secure (type B), anxious-avoidant (Type A), and anxious-resistant (Type C) children, these children consistently lacked organized strategies for dealing with stressful separations from and reunions with their caregiver. Main and Solomon described this pattern of attachment as "disorganized–disoriented" (Type D). In addition, these children displayed other bizarre symptoms in the presence of their caregiver such as interrupted movements and expressions, freezing and stilling behaviors, and apprehension (Main and Solomon 1986). See Table 1 for a summary of the behavioral organization characteristics of each of the four major patterns of attachment.

Recent investigations of attachment in maltreated infants and toddlers indicate a preponderance of atypical attachment patterns in maltreated children. Carlson, Cicchetti, Barnett, and Braunwald (1989) found that over 80% of the maltreated infants in their study had atypical, disorganized/disoriented attachments compared to less than 20% of a demographically similar nonmaltreated comparison groups. Similar findings have been reported by Lyons-Ruth, Repacholi, McLeod, and Silva (1991). Crittenden (1988) found in her study that most maltreated children could be classified as having avoidant-ambivalent (A-C) patterns of attachment. Recently, there have been findings of substantial stability in one of the forms of atypical attachment across the ages of 12,

Table 1

PATTERNS OF CHILDREN'S INTERACTIVE BEHAVIOR WITH THE
CAREGIVER IN THE STRANGE SITUATION ASSOCIATED WITH
THE FOUR MAJOR ATTACHMENT CLASSIFICATIONS

	Patterns of Attachment	Description of Interactive Behaviors
Type A	Anxious–avoidant	*Independent exploration* (e.g., readily separates to explore during preseparation; little affective sharing; affiliative to stranger). *Active avoidance upon reunion* (e.g., turning away, looking away, moving away, ignoring; no avoidance of stranger).
Type B	Secure	*Caregiver is a secure base for exploration* (e.g., readily separates to explore toys; affective sharing of play; affiliative to stranger in mother's presence; readily comforted when distressed). *Active in seeking contact or interaction upon reunion* (e.g., if distressed, immediately seek and maintain contact, and contact is effective in terminating distress; if not distressed, active greeting behavior and strong initiation of interaction.
Type C	Anxious–Resistant	*Poverty of exploration* (e.g., difficulty separating to explore; may need contact even prior to separation; wary of novel situations and people). *Difficulty settling upon reunion* (e.g., may mix contact seeking with contact resistance such as hitting and kicking; may continue to cry and fuss; may show noticeable passivity).
Type D	Disorganized/disoriented	*Sequential and/or simultaneous displays of contradictory behavior patterns; undirected and incomplete movements and expressions; stereotypies; asymmetrical movements; anomalous postures; freezing, stilling, and dazing; apprehension toward caregiver.*

Adapted from Ainsworth, Blehar, Waters, and Wall (1978); and from Main and Solomon (1990).

18, and 24 months. Barnett, Ganiban, and Cicchetti (1991) found that approximately 60% of the infants who were classified as D at 12 months had the same classification at 24 months, while over 90% of the infants classified as D at 24 months had previously received the D classification.

As children grow older, though, it appears less certain that they will have one of these atypical patterns of attachment. In an investigation of the attachments of maltreated preschool children of different ages (Cicchetti & Barnett, 1991a), 30-month-old children who had been maltreated were significantly more likely to have atypical patterns of attachment ("D" or "A/C") than were nonmaltreated children. However, even though approximately one third of the 36-month-old and

48-month-old maltreated children had either Type D or A/C attachments, this was not significantly greater than the proportion of nonmaltreated children who had such atypical attachment patterns. Along these lines, Lynch and Cicchetti (1991) found that approximately 30% of maltreated children between the ages of 7 and 13 years reported having "confused" patterns of relatedness to their mothers. This finding suggests that distortions in maltreated children's relationships with and mental representations of their caregivers may persist up through the preadolescent years, though at lower rates than found in early infancy.

There are several possible explanations for the apparent decline in disorganized and other atypical attachment patterns at older ages. It is conceivable that the attachment coding system for preschool children (Cassidy and Marvin 1991) may utilize overly conservative criteria for detecting disorganization in the attachments of older children. It also is possible that older children represent their maltreating attachment relationship in ways that are organized differently than the representations of younger children. Cognitive maturity may play a role in how children are able to represent maltreating relationships and themselves in such relationships, and how they are able to organize their attachment behavior strategies. Disorganization may be a characteristic feature of less differentiated and integrated mental representations and strategies. Severity, chronicity, and type of abuse, as well as specific maltreatment history, probably interact with cognitive maturity in determining the nature of mental representation also. It is clear that many important questions regarding the manner in which relationship experiences and cognitive maturity interact as determinants of mental representation remain to be answered.

These questions notwithstanding, the findings on the prevalence and stability of insecure and atypical attachments in maltreated children point to the extreme risk these children face in achieving adaptive outcomes in other domains of interpersonal relationships. Internal representational models of these insecure and often atypical attachments, with their complementary models of self and other, may generalize to new relationships, leading to negative expectations of how others will behave and how successful the self will be in relation to others.

Another important task of early ontogenic development is emotion regulation (Cicchetti 1990b). Maltreated children have been shown to have deficits in their emotional self-regulation (Cicchetti, Ganiban, and Barnett 1991). As a result, both the modulation and initiation of positive and negative affect can be problematic for these children. Gaensbauer and his colleagues (Gaensbauer and Hiatt 1984;

Gaensbaurer, Mrazek, and Harmon 1980) have observed distortions in the initial patterns of affect differentiation in maltreated infants. They appear to exhibit either excessive amounts of negative affect or, in contrast, blunted patterns of affect where they express neither positive nor negative emotions. In addition to problems in the differentiation of emotional expression, maltreated children also have difficulty processing emotional stimuli. Camras has found that maltreated children are less able to decode facial expressions of emotion than nonmaltreated comparison children (Camras, Grow, and Ribordy 1983).

Emotion regulation may also play a role in the disorganization found in maltreated children's attachment relationships. The fear that is elicited in these relationships may paralyze or severely impair maltreated children's ability to regulate and organize their affects. In fact, maltreated children exhibit a profile of symptoms similar to that of individuals suffering from chronic stress including anxiety, low tolerance to stress, depression, and helplessness (Kazdin, Moser, Colbus, and Bell 1985; Wolfe 1985). The loss of the attachment figure as a secure base and haven of safety is a devastating psychological insult and may lead to long-term psychobiological impairments such as those found in posttraumatic stress disorder (Cicchetti, Ganiban, and Barnett 1991; van der Kolk 1987).

In the context of child maltreatment, it is important to realize that caregivers can exert a major impact on the socialization of affect. The types of affect a child is capable of expressing; the range, intensity, and duration of affective expression; the contexts in which emotions are expressed; and the regulation of emotional displays — all are areas that can be affected by parental socialization (Cicchetti and Schneider-Rosen 1984, 1986). By examining this process of socialization, we have access to how features of the child's microsystem influence ontogenic development. Parental use of internal-state language is one such area that can add to our understanding of the development of emotion regulation (Bretherton and Beeghly 1982).

It has been suggested that the use of emotion language helps one control non-verbal emotional expressions, which in turn enhances regulation of the emotions themselves (Hesse and Cicchetti 1982). Thus, parents who frequently use emotional language to interpret nonverbal emotional expressions may provide their children with mechanisms that help control their own emotional expressions. In contrast, parents who use emotion language to intellectualize or defend against emotional experience may be exhibiting an overcontrolled coping style. One can argue then, that parents transfer their coping skills to their children through their use of emotional language (Hesse and Cicchetti 1982). Consistent with this view is the finding that maltreated toddlers lag behind nonmaltreated children in their use of internal-state words about the self and others (Cicchetti and Beeghly 1987).

Some of the coping skills that maltreated children acquire can be seen in the types of cognitive control functioning that they use in service of emotional self-regulation. Cognitive controls are viewed as coordinating the requirements of external stimuli with those of internal fantasies and affects (Santostefano 1978, 1985). Rieder and Cicchetti (1989) have found that maltreated children are more distracted by aggressive stimuli and recall a greater number of distracting aggressive stimuli than do nonmaltreated children. Maltreated children assimilate aggressive stimuli more readily, even though this may result in less cognitive efficiency and impaired task performance. Originally, hypervigilance and ready assimilation of aggressive stimuli may have developed as an adaptive coping strategy in the maltreating environment, alerting the child to signs of imminent danger and keeping affects from rising so high that they would incapacitate the child. This strategy may also be helpful to the child in identifying specific elements of the current situation in an effort to determine the most adaptive response. However, this response pattern becomes less adaptive when the child is faced with nonthreatening situations and may even undermine the child's ability to function adaptively under normal circumstances. We suggest that the poor-quality representational models of attachment figures and of the self that maltreated children develop early in life predispose them to manifest these impairments in information processing and in cognitive control function.

The development of an autonomous self is yet another important issue of ontogenic development (Cicchetti 1990b). Again we can see how the microsystem impacts maltreated children's ontogenesis. Knowing that maltreated children receive chronically insensitive care from their parents (Crittenden 1981; Trickett and Sussman 1988) and that they are likely to experience insecure attachment relationships, one would expect that maltreated children's sense of self might be impaired. Existing research substantiates this claim with regard to maltreated children's self-concept and self-esteem.

In visual self-recognition experiments, maltreated toddlers are more likely than comparison children to express either neutral or negative affect when viewing their rouge-marked faces in the mirror (Schneider-Rosen and Cicchetti 1984, 1991), possibly indicating an early precursor to a generalized low sense of self-worth. In another study of self-differentiation in maltreated toddlers, Egeland and Sroufe (1981) employed a tool-use/problem-solving paradigm to investigate 24-month-old children's emerging autonomy, independent exploration, and ability to cope with frustration. They found that maltreated children become more angry, frustrated with mother, and noncompliant than comparison children do, suggesting that maltreated children at this age have difficulty making a smooth transition toward autonomy. Other delays in the development of self-systems have been noted above, such as the finding that maltreated toddlers talk less about themselves and produce less internal-state language than do comparison toddlers (Cicchetti and Beeghly

1987; Coster, Gersten, Beeghly, and Cicchetti 1989).

Finally, Vondra, Barnett, and Cicchetti (1989, 1990) found that young maltreated children (grades 1–3) see themselves as being more competent and accepted than comparison children do, and also as more competent than their teachers believe them to be. It is possible that these young maltreated children's inflated self-perceptions reflect unrealistic coping strategies that help them gain a sense of personal competence and control in home settings that are chaotic and uncontrollable. In contrast, though, older maltreated children describe themselves as less competent and accepted than comparison children do, and more in accordance with teacher ratings. It may be the case that the older children's ability to make social comparisons causes them to make more accurate appraisals of themselves than younger maltreated children, resulting in feelings of generalized low self-worth.

Another important task of ontogenic development is the formation of effective peer relations (Cicchetti 1990b). Because of their frequently negative relationship histories, peer relationships and friendships may play an especially important role in promoting positive adaptation in maltreated children (Cicchetti, Lynch, Shonk, and Todd Manly 1992). Many important issues of social and emotional development are facilitated by children exposed to the social world of peers (Hartup 1983). Consequently, poor peer relationships have been associated with juvenile delinquency and other types of behavior disorders (Rutter and Giller 1983). Unfortunately, several studies indicate that maltreated children are at risk for developing poor peer relationships. Positive, secure family relationships have been associated with adaptive, competent peer relationships, while atypical, insecure family relationships are associated with less competent and sometimes maladaptive peer relationships (Sroufe and Fleeson 1986; Troy and Sroufe 1987).

In general, the literature suggests that maltreated children display more disturbed patterns of interaction with their peers than do nonmaltreated children. They interact less with their peers and exhibit less prosocial behavior (Hoffman-Plotkin and Twentyman 1984; Jacobson and Straker 1982). If maltreated children's representational models of others reflect insecurity and fear based on their attachment histories with their caregivers (Crittenden and Ainsworth 1989), they may enter relationships with new social partners such as peers with approach/avoidance conflicts that result in maladaptive patterns of relating. Alternatively, the fear incorporated into many maltreated children's models could lead to both "flight" and "fight" responses toward potential social partners (Cicchetti, Lynch et al. 1992). From an organizational/relationship perspective, where an individual's self-organization is determined by his or her relationship history (Sroufe 1989), this flight-or-fight pattern would be observed in maltreated children if they internalize both sides of their relationship with their caregiver (i.e., being both the victim and the victimizer – see Troy and Sroufe 1987). As a result, maltreated children may end up alternately avoiding others and being aggressive toward them.

Consistent with this hypothesis, Mueller and Silverman (1989) have identified two main themes in the findings on maltreated children's peer relationships. One, maltreated children, especially physically abused children, tend to show heightened levels of physical and verbal aggression in their interactions with peers (George and Main 1979; Hoffman-Plotkin and Twentyman 1984; Kaufman and Cicchetti 1989). Two, there is a high degree of withdrawal from and avoidance of peer interactions in maltreated children as compared to nonmaltreated children (George and Main 1979; Hoffman-Plotkin and Twentyman 1984; Howes and Espinosa 1985; Jacobson and Straker 1982). Overall, Mueller and Silverman (1989) conclude that the heightened aggressiveness, avoidance, and aberrant responses to both friendly overtures and distress in peers suggest that maltreated children are unprepared to develop successful peer relationships. Instead, contact with peers seems to elicit stressful reactions from maltreated children that decrease the likelihood of further interaction (Mueller and Silverman 1989).

One final example of a central task of ontogenic development is successful adaptation to school (Cicchetti 1990b). Integration into the peer group, acceptable performance in the classroom, and appropriate motivational orientations for achievement all are part of this stage-salient developmental task. Once again, however, maltreated children appear to be at risk for an unsuccessful resolution to this issue of development. Eckenrode and Laird (1991) report that maltreated children perform lower on standardized tests and obtain worse grades than nonmaltreated children do while receiving more referrals and suspensions for discipline problems. Other investigators have found that maltreated children are dependent on their teachers (Egeland, Sroufe, and Erickson 1983); score lower on tests measuring cognitive maturity, perhaps because of motivational reasons (Barahal, Waterman, and Martin, 1981); and are rated by both parents and teachers as less ready to learn in school (Hoffman-Plotkin and Twentyman, 1984).

An especially important factor in resolving the task of adaptation to school may be secure readiness to learn. Aber and Allen (1987) proposed that effectance motivation, which is the intrinsic desire to deal competently with one's environment, and successful relations with novel adults (i.e., relations that are characterized neither by dependency nor wariness) are important components of children being able to adapt to their first major out-of-home environment. Secure readiness to learn is characterized by high effectance motivation and low dependency. Maltreated children consistently score lower than comparison groups of children on a secure readiness to learn factor (Aber and Allen 1987; Aber, Allen, Carlson, and Cicchetti 1989). Secure readiness to learn appears to represent a dynamic balance between establish-ing secure relationships with adults and feeling free to explore the environment in ways that will promote cognitive competence. The findings of Aber and his colleagues are particularly compelling because they are congruent with prior research on how maltreatment affects infants' and toddlers' development. At both of these developmental stages, maltreatment interferes with the balance between the motivation to establish secure relationships with adults and the motivation to explore the world in competency-promoting ways.

Behavior Problems and Psychopathology

As we have seen, maltreated children display disturbed functioning on each of the stage-salient issues of early development. Specifically, dysfunctional attachment relationships and representational models of the self and others, difficulties in emotional self-regulation, deviations in self-system processes, problematic peer relationships, and trouble adapting to school were found in maltreated children. These repeated developmental disruptions create a profile of vulnerability factors that places maltreated children at high risk for future maladaptation. Although not all maltreated children who have trouble resolving stage-salient issues will develop psychopathology, let alone the same form of pathology, later disturbances in functioning are likely to occur (Cicchetti 1990b). A number of research findings are relevant to understanding how behavior problems and psychopathology may emerge according to an ecological/transactional model.

Aber, Allen, Carlson, and Cicchetti (1989) examined the relation between parent-reported symptoms on the Achenbach Child Behavior Checklist (Achenbach and Edelbrock 1983) and the two constructs of secure readiness to learn and outer-directedness, which has been defined as an orientation to problem solving in which children rely on external cues rather than their own cognitive resources. They found no difference between maltreated and nonmaltreated comparison preschool children in levels of parent-reported symptoms. There were, however, clear associations between symptoms and the two developmental variables. Low secure readiness to learn predicted social withdrawal, aggression, and depression in *maltreated* preschoolers, and high outer-directedness predicted social withdrawal and aggression in *nonmaltreated* comparison preschoolers.

These findings of different developmental correlates of symptomatology for maltreated and nonmaltreated preschool children may reflect children's adaptation to the specific parenting styles of maltreating parents. For example, Crittenden (1988) has observed maltreated preschool children's compulsive compliance to their parents' excessive demands. This may foster outer-directedness in maltreated children. On the other hand, Main and Goldwyn (1984) have noted that maltreating parents have unrealistically high expectations of independence and autonomy for their children, and they become upset by their children's dependency needs. Thus, maltreating parents may themselves associate low secure readiness with problems in their children while they continue to foster an orientation of outer-directedness in their children, which is contrary to secure readiness. The results of differential developmental correlates of symptomatology suggest that although lower-SES maltreated and nonmaltreated children appear equally depressed, withdrawn, and aggressive, there may be different underlying developmental pathways that account for similar patterns in the phenotypic expression of symptoms (*cf.* Cicchetti and Schneider-Rosen 1986). Maltreated preschoolers may become symptomatic through a pathway of low secure readiness to learn. Nonmaltreated preschoolers may become symptomatic through a pathway of high outer-directedness (Aber et al. 1989). These different developmental pathways and processes appear to be congruent with differences in microsystemic child-rearing styles and family ecologies.

In contrast to the findings for preschoolers, maltreated children were significantly more depressed and socially withdrawn as well as marginally more aggressive than nonmaltreated children during the early school years. Comparing these data with norms for clinic-referred and nonclinical samples of children indicated that maltreated children scored within the clinical range in symptoms. Two recent studies support these findings. Toth, Manly, and Cicchetti (1992) found that physically abused children between the ages of 7 and 12 years evidenced significantly more depressive symptomatology than children from either neglectful or nonmaltreating families. In addition, physically abused children exhibited the lowest levels of self-esteem. These findings point to the particularly damaging effects of physical abuse on children's self-development and emotional adaptation.

Additionally, in a study that investigated the effects of various types of domestic violence on children's behavior problems and depression, Sternberg, Lamb, and their colleagues found that children who had been physically abused reported higher levels of problematic behavior and depression than did children who had witnessed spouse abuse or who had experienced no known domestic violence (Sternberg et al. in press). Moreover, according to their mothers, children who had witnessed spouse abuse had higher levels of problematic behavior (Sternberg et al. in press). The results of this study demonstrate that domestic violence has effects on child development that vary in nature depending on the type of domestic violence and the source of information about the child's adjustment.

CONCLUSION

In this paper, we have outlined a model that provides an explanatory framework for understanding the causes and consequences of community violence and child maltreatment for individuals, families, and communities. By examining each level of our ecological/transactional model, we begin to see the pathways by which violence in its multiple forms acts as a potentiating factor for adverse developmental outcomes in children. We offer several prescriptions for future investigations of the etiology and sequelae of community violence and child maltreatment.

First, further specification and operationalization of each of the levels of the model is required. Effort should be made to identify the factors that properly define each level of the ecological model so that they can be measured and examined. Particular attention needs to be given to defining features of the macro- and exosystems that are relevant to the study of community violence and child maltreatment. Once the model's nested levels are specified, links across levels will be easier to identify. Rather than solely studying factors at a single level of the model and their relationships to outcome variables, we should be seeking to uncover transactions that occur among levels and the ways in which these intersystemic interplays mediate the effects of each other on children's adaptation. For example, the presence of violence at one level of the model does not necessarily condemn children to poor developmental outcomes. The existence of pervasive community violence is a feature of the exosystem that can act as a potentiating factor for the occurrence of violence within the family. However, other components of the microsystem such as maternal education and secure parental attachment histories can act as compensatory factors against the occurrence of familial violence, thus functioning as enduring protective factors in children's overall adaptation. Here we see mediational effects across levels of the ecological/transactional model that would explain resilient outcomes for some children exposed to community violence. At all levels of the model, potentiating and compensatory risk factors are operating. It is the transactions among ecological levels that result in potentiating and compensatory factors and in mechanisms for the precursors and sequelae of community violence and child maltreatment.

A more precise understanding of the operation of risk factors within the model is needed, however. In particular, it is important to consider that factors that increase or decrease the likelihood of risk during one period of children's development may not do so during other developmental periods. Moreover, the temporal dimension of potentiating and compensatory risk factors is not static. Risk factors that were enduring can become transient, and vice versa. For example, potentiators that originally are associated with relatively transient factors, such as initial unemployment, can become enduring when they persist over time, as in the case of chronic unemployment. It is even possible that risk factors that had acted as potentiators can be associated later on with compensatory risk factors. Perhaps the successful handling of a challenge can result in the development of new compensatory factors. For example, children who are able to survive the direct and indirect challenges presented by such potentiating factors as poverty, community violence, or child maltreatment may develop inner characteristics that later are able to function as compensatory factors. The reverse is also possible. A compensatory risk factor could become a potentiating risk factor for maladaptation. As a result, adding a developmental perspective to conceptualizations of risk is necessary to specify how potentiating and compensatory risk factors operate within the model.

In addition, violence itself needs to be defined more clearly. Researchers in the area of child maltreatment have had to accept this challenge (cf. Cicchetti 1991). Maltreatment is a heterogeneous phenomenon that has a broad range of manifestations, some of which include violence. In addition to indicating the type or types of maltreatment that are occurring, it is important to specify how severe the maltreatment is, how long it has been occurring, who the perpetrator is, and how old the child is (Cicchetti and Barnett 1991b). Investigators of the causes and consequences of community violence should make similar attempts at clearly defining specific types of violence. They should go beyond the use of crime statistics and self-reports as their chief indicators of the incidence and prevalence of violence in the community and in the family. One important direction for future research will be the development and validation of a nosology for classifying community violence. It is clear that violence encompasses a broad range of phenomena that have varying manifestations and that operate in different ecological systems. Currently, however, there is no accepted system for classifying these diverse experiences. Consequently, the interpretation of research findings across laboratories and the assessment of intervention efficacy is much more difficult. A comprehensive violence classification system could provide researchers and clinicians from different disciplines with a uniform method of assessing important information and communicating with one another. Such a system would enable investigators to determine the processes by which violence occurs and the differential impact that a variety of violent experiences have on children at different points in their development.

Another necessary step is to integrate epidemiological approaches to the study of community violence and child maltreatment with direct observational, interview, and experimental procedures. Now that epidemiologists possess excellent techniques for selecting representative samples of these target populations, it is possible to choose a random subsample of a larger representative group of families and individuals to study more intensively. In this vein, studies could be conducted that examine the direct and indirect effects of community violence on children and families. From an ecological/transactional perspective, it will be critical to assess the mediators of these effects from different ecological systems. For example, issues such as whether the children in the family are being maltreated, spouse abuse is occurring, the family is satisfied with its social networks and neighborhood sup-

ports, and the spousal and family relationships are harmonious all could influence the links from community violence to child and family functioning. We believe that the time has come to initiate multidisciplinary collaborative research projects on the effects of community violence and child maltreatment. Furthermore, such studies should be carried out in multiple contexts concurrently (e.g., the home, research laboratories, community settings, etc.).

Moreover, research on the causes and consequences of community violence and child maltreatment should be implemented with a lifespan developmental perspective as the guiding framework. Thus, investigators must strive to ascertain a complete and accurate historical and contemporary portrayal of all forms of violence each participant in their investigations has experienced. As a result, researchers would be in a position to examine the links between community violence and child maltreatment. In addition, this lifespan approach, in concert with efforts to develop a scientifically valid nosology, would provide us with an initial understanding of how violence in all of its forms is transmitted across generations in differing community and family contexts.

A research agenda that proposes a systematic inquiry into the effects of community violence is needed. Important questions to address concern the long-term consequences of exposure to chronic violence, and characteristics of communities, families, and individuals that mediate reactions to community violence. There is much to be learned about how exposure to violence affects children's views of the world and of themselves, their investment in and ability to form stable relationships, and their ability to experience and modulate arousal (Cicchetti, Ganiban, and Barnett 1991; Ornitz and Pynoos 1989; Terr 1991; van der Kolk 1987). In addition, it is important that we understand the risk factors, both potentiating and compensatory, that are associated with experiencing different amounts and types of violence.

It is along these lines that an ecological/

transactional model of community violence and child maltreatment may be most helpful. The presence of community violence and child maltreatment both undoubtedly act as potentiators of negative developmental outcomes for children. Moreover, the presence or absence of either community violence or child maltreatment may influence the effects of the other. An ecological/transactional model suggests to us questions that need to be addressed to understand the effects of community violence and child maltreatment. Studies need to be conducted that assess the independent effects of community violence and child maltreatment on children's development. How community violence influences development in the absence of child maltreatment, and vice versa, are important questions to answer. Furthermore, we need studies that examine the interaction between community violence and child maltreatment and their combined effect on child outcomes. By investigating the processes involved in such interactions, it will be possible to answer such questions as whether the absence of child maltreatment is a compensatory risk factor for the effect of community violence on children's adaptation. Moreover, the absence of community violence may be a compensatory risk factor for the effects of child maltreatment. Currently, such studies on the effects of community violence and child maltreatment are being conducted in our laboratory.

Finally, we have suggested that the representational models of attachment figures and of the self in relation to others that individuals develop in the course of relating with their primary caregivers may be one mechanism for perpetuating violence across generations. Similarly, since these representational models are carried forward into other relationships, they may provide one possible means whereby people re-create or perpetuate their earlier violent experiences. Because individuals internalize whole relationships, it is not uncommon to observe victims of violence within families victimizing other family members. It is also possible that acts of violence and aggres-

sion become internalized as generalized response patterns (Rieder and Cicchetti 1989). Thus, when children who have been exposed to violence encounter interpersonal situations and they access their corresponding representational models, they may be more likely to activate an aggressive behavioral response pattern, whether or not it is appropriate (see Main and George 1985; Kaufman and Cicchetti 1989; Troy and Sroufe 1987). For example, the exploiter–exploited relationships that maltreated children engage in with their parents often take other forms such as when a physically abused child becomes hostile toward a peer partner (Troy & Sroufe 1987). Moreover, some maltreated children have been observed to respond to peers who are in distress with comforting behaviors. However, their initial comforting response then escalates into an aggressive attack on the distressed peer (Main and George 1985).

In a related vein, Reiss (1981) has described family paradigms as the set of core assumptions, beliefs, or convictions that families hold about their environment. Reiss contends that these paradigms affect how families process information about the world. Similar to individual representational models, Reiss states that these family paradigms are relatively enduring and that these core beliefs develop in the course of family development (cf. Cicchetti and Howes, 1991). We suggest that these family paradigms may be conceptualized as the family's representational model of the community in which they reside. We believe that these "community" models may be one mechanism for perpetuating violence in communities. For example, they may shape the individual's expectations of how the community will treat him or her as well as what the individual's own place is within the broader community. Likewise, these models may shape families' viewpoints and expectations surrounding their role and value in the community. Of course, there most likely are interactions between the quality of children's representational models of relationships and the nature of family representational models of the community that parents encourage. We think that this is a ripe area for future theorizing and research. From the perspective of the ecological/transactional model proposed herein, we suggest that the negative expectations that accompany the representational models of children and families experiencing and being exposed to violence may result in the perpetuation of violence both across generations and throughout all levels of ecological systems.

We believe that the model of community violence and child maltreatment that we have proposed provides a framework that will help prevention and intervention efforts to target areas of need. The model suggests that work may need to be carried out at different levels of the ecology in order to ameliorate the effects of community violence and child maltreatment. Clearly, as our ecological/transactional approach indicates, there are no simple solutions or correctives that can be applied to the causes and consequences of community violence and child maltreatment. Rather, the implication of this model is that far-reaching social policies are needed that will address all levels of children's ecologies.

REFERENCES

ABER, J. L., and ALLEN, J. P. The effects of maltreatment on young children's socio-emotional development: An attachment theory perspective. *Developmental Psychology* (1987) 23:406–14.

ABER, J. L., ALLEN, J., CARLSON, V., and CICCHETTI, D. The effects of maltreatment on development during early childhood: Recent studies and their theoretical, clinical, and policy implications. In D. Cicchetti and V. Carlson, eds., *Child Maltreatment: Theory and Research on the Causes and Consequences of Child Abuse and Neglect.* Cambridge University Press, 1989.

ACHENBACH, T. M., and EDELBROCK, C. S. *Manual for the Child Behavior Checklist and Revised Child Behavior Profile.* University of Vermont Department of Psychiatry, 1983.

AINSWORTH, M. D. S., BLEHAR, M. C., WATERS, E., and WALL, S. *Patterns of Attachment: A Psychological Study of the Strange Situation.* Lawrence Erlbaum Associates, 1978.

ALTEMEIER, W., O'CONNER, S., VIETZE, P., SANDLER, H., and SHERROD, K. Antecedents of child abuse. *Journal of Pediatrics* (1982) 100:823–29.

BARAHAL, R., WATERMAN, J., and MARTIN, H. The social-cognitive development of abused children. *Journal of Consulting and Clinical Psychology* (1981) 49:508–16.

BARNETT, D., GANIBAN, J., and CICCHETTI, D. *Temperament and behavior of youngsters with disorganized attachments.* Manuscript submitted for publication, 1991.

BELSKY, J. Child maltreatment: An ecological integration. *American Psychologist* (1980) 35:320–35.

BELSKY, J. The determinants of parenting: A process model. *Child Development* (1984) 55:83–96.

BOWLBY, J. *Attachment and Loss*, Vol. 1. Basic Books, 1969/1982.

BOWLBY, J. *Attachment and Loss: Loss, Sadness, and Depression.* Basic Books, 1980.

BRETHERTON, I., and BEEGHLY, M. Talking about internal states: The acquisition of an explicit theory of mind. *Developmental Psychology* (1982) 18: 906–21.

BRONFENBRENNER, U. Toward an experimental ecology of human development. *American Psychologist* (1977) 32:513–31.

BRUNQUELL, D., CRICHTON, L., and EGELAND, B. Maternal personality and attitude in disturbances of child rearing. *American Journal of Orthopsychiatry* (1981) 51:680–90.

BUREAU OF JUSTICE STATISTICS. *Report to the Nation on Crime and Justice: The Data.* Department of Justice, 1983.

BURGESS, R., and CONGER, R. Family interaction of abusive, neglectful and normal families. *Child Development* (1978) 49:1163–73.

CAMRAS, L., GROW, J. G., and RIBORDY, S. Recognition of emotional expression by abused children. *Journal of Clinical Child Psychology* (1983) 12: 325–28.

CARLSON, V., CICCHETTI, D., BARNETT, D., and BRAUNWALD, K. Disorganized/disoriented attachment relationships in maltreated infants. *Developmental Psychopathology* (1989) 25:525–31.

CASSIDY, J., and MARVIN, R. S. *Attachment Organization in Three- and Four-Year Olds: Coding Guidelines.* Pennsylvania State University and the University of Virginia, 1991.

CHRISTOFFEL, K. K. Violent death and injury in US children and adolescents. *American Journal of Disease Control* (1990) 144:697–706.

CICCHETTI, D. How research on child maltreatment has informed the study of child development: Perspectives from developmental psychopathology. In D. Cicchetti and V. Carlson, eds., *Child Maltreatment: Theory and Research on the Causes and Consequences of Child Abuse and Neglect.* Cambridge University Press, 1989.

CICCHETTI, D. Developmental psychopathology and the prevention of serious mental disorders: Overdue detente and illustrations through the affective disorders. In P. Muehrer, ed., *Conceptual Re-*

search Models for Prevention of Mental Disorders, NIMH, 1990a.

CICCHETTI, D. The organization and coherence of socioemotional, cognitive, and representational development: Illustrations through a developmental psychopathology perspective on Down syndrome and child maltreatment. In R. Thompson, ed., *Nebraska Symposium on Motivation*, Vol. 36: *Socioemotional Development*. University of Nebraska Press, 1990b.

CICCHETTI, D., ed. Special issue: Defining psychological maltreatment. *Development and Psychopathology* (1991) 3(1).

CICCHETTI, D., and BARNETT, D. Attachment organization in maltreated preschoolers. *Development and Psychopathology* (1991a) 3:397–411.

CICCHETTI, D., and BARNETT, D. Toward the development of a scientific nosology of child maltreatment. In D. Cicchetti and W. Grove, eds., *Thinking Clearly About Psychology: Essays in Honor of Paul E. Meehl*, Vol. 2: *Personality and Psychopathology*. University of Minnesota Press, 1991b.

CICCHETTI, C., and BEEGHLY, M. Symbolic development in maltreated youngsters: An organizational perspective. *New Directions for Child Development* (1987) 36:5–29.

CICCHETTI, D., and CARLSON, V., eds. *Child Maltreatment: Theory and Research on the Causes and Consequences of Child Abuse and Neglect*. Cambridge University Press, 1989.

CICCHETTI, D., CUMMINGS, M., GREENBERG, M., and MARVIN, R. Attachment beyond infancy. In M. Greenberg, D. Cicchetti, and M. Cummings, eds., *Attachment During the Preschool Years*. University of Chicago Press, 1990.

CICCHETTI, D., GANIBAN, J., and BARNETT, D. Contributions from the Study of High Risk Populations to Understanding the Development of Emotion Regulation. In K. Dodge and J. Garber, eds., *The Development of Emotion Regulation*. Cambridge University Press, 1991.

CICCHETTI, D., and HOWES, P. W. Developmental psychopathology in the context of the family: Illustrations from the study of child maltreatment. *Canadian Journal of Behavioural Science* (1991) 23:257–81.

CICCHETTI, D., LYNCH, M., SHONK, S., and TODD MANLY, J. An organizational perspective on peer relations in maltreated children. In R. D. Parke and G. W. Ladd, eds., *Family-Peer Relationships: Modes of Linkage*. Lawrence Erlbaum Associates, 1992.

CICCHETTI, D., and RIZLEY, R. Developmental perspectives on the etiology, intergenerational transmission, and sequelae of child maltreatment. *New Directions for Child Development* (1981) 11:31–55.

CICCHETTI, D., and SCHNEIDER-ROSEN, L. Theoretical and empirical considerations in the investigation of the relationships between effect and cognition in atypical populations of infants: Contributions to the formulation of an integrative theory of development. In C. Izard, J. Kagan, and R. Zajonc, eds., *Emotions, Cognition and Behavior*. Cambridge University Press, 1984.

CICCHETTI, D., and SCHNEIDER-ROSEN, K. An organizational approach to childhood depression. In M. Rutter, C. Izard, and P. Read, eds., *Depression in Young People: Clinical and Developmental Perspectives*. Guilford Press, 1986.

CONGER, R., BURGESS, R., and BARRETT, C. Child abuse related to life change and perceptions of illness: Some preliminary findings. *Family Coordinator* (1979) 28:73–78.

CORSE, S., SCHMID, K., and TRICKETT, P. Social network characteristics of mothers in abusing and non-abusing families and their relationships to parenting beliefs. *Journal of Community Psychology* (1990) 18:44–59.

COSTER, W. J., GERSTEN, M. S., BEEGHLY, M., and CICCHETTI, D. Communicative functioning in maltreated toddlers. *Developmental Psychology* (1989) 25:1020–29.

CRITTENDEN, P. M. Abusing, neglecting, problematic, and adequate dyads: Differentiating by patterns of interaction. *Merrill-Palmer Quarterly* (1981) 27:201–08.

CRITTENDEN, P. M. Social networks, quality of parenting, and child development. *Child Development* (1985) 56:1299–1313.

CRITTENDEN, P. M. Distorted patterns of relationship in maltreating families: The role of internal representational models. *Journal of Reproductive and Infant Psychology* (1988) 6:183–99.

CRITTENDEN, P., and AINSWORTH, M. Attachment and child abuse. In D. Cicchetti and V. Carlson, eds., *Child maltreatment: Theory and Research on the Causes and Consequences of Child Abuse and Neglect*. Cambridge University Press, 1989.

DEAN, A., MALIK, M., RICHARDS, W., and STRINGER, S. Effects of parental maltreatment on children's conceptions of interpersonal relationships. *Developmental Psychology* (1986) 22:617–26.

ECKENRODE, J., and LAIRD, M. *Social adjustment of maltreated children in the school setting*. Paper presented at the biennial meeting of the Society for Research in Child Development, Seattle, WA, 1991.

EGELAND, B., and BRUNQUELL, D. An at-risk approach to the study of child abuse: Some preliminary findings. *Journal of the American Academy of Child Psychiatry* (1979) 18:219–35.

EGELAND, B., and SROUFE, L. A. Developmental sequelae of maltreatment in infancy. *New Directions for Child Development* (1981) 11:77–92.

EGELAND, B., JACOBVITZ, D., and PAPATOLA, K. Intergenerational continuity of abuse. In R. J. Gelles and J. B. Lancaster, eds., *Child Abuse and Neglect: Biosocial Dimensions*. Aldine, 1987.

EGELAND, B., SROUFE, L. A., and ERICKSON, M. The developmental consequence of different patterns of maltreatment. *Child Abuse and Neglect* (1983) 7:459–69.

ERICKSON, M. F., EGELAND, B., and PIANTA, R. The effects of maltreatment on the development of young children. In D. Cicchetti and V. Carlson, eds., *Child Maltreatment: Theory and Research on the Causes and Consequences of Child Abuse and Neglect*. Cambridge University Press, 1989.

FESHBACH, S. The development and regulation of aggression: Some research gaps and a proposed cognitive analysis. In J. DeWitt and W. Hartup, eds., *Determinants and Origins of Aggressive Behavior.* Mouton, 1974.

FINGERHUT, L. A., and KLEINMAN, J. C. International and interstate comparisons of homicide among young males. *Journal of the American Medical Association.* (1990) 263:3292–95.

GAENSBAUER, T. J., and HIATT, S. Facial communication of emotion in early infancy. In N. A. Fox and R. J. Davidson, eds., *The Psychobiology of Affective Development.* Lawrence Erlbaum Associates, 1984.

GAENSBAUER, T., MRAZEK, D., and HARMON, R. Affective behavior patterns in abused and/or neglected infants. In N. Freud, ed., *The Understanding and Prevention of Child Abuse: Psychological Approaches.* Concord Press, 1980.

GARBARINO, J. A preliminary study of some ecological correlates of child abuse: The impact of socioeconomic stress on mothers. *Child Development* (1976) 57:372–81.

GARBARINO, J. The human ecology of child maltreatment: A conceptual model for research. *Journal of Marriage and the Family* (1977) 39:721–32.

GARBARINO, J. *Children and Families in the Social Environment.* Aldine, 1982.

GARBARINO, J., and GILLIAM, G. *Understanding Abusive Families.* Lexington Press, 1980.

GARBARINO, J., GUTTMANN, E., and SEELEY, J. *The Psychologically Battered Child.* Jossey-Bass, 1986.

GARBARINO, J., and KOSTELNY, K. *Child Maltreatment as a Community Problem.* Submitted for publication, 1991.

GARBARINO, J., KOSTELNY, K., and DUBROW, N. What children can tell us about living in danger. *American Psychologist* (1991) 46:376–83.

GARBARINO, J., and SHERMAN, D. High-risk neighborhoods and high-risk families: The human ecology of child maltreatment. *Child Development* (1980) 51:188–98.

GEORGE, C., and MAIN, M. Social interactions of young abused children: Approach, avoidance, and aggression. *Child Development* (1979) 50:306–18.

GIL, D. *Violence Against Children: Physical Child Abuse in the United States.* Harvard University Press, 1970.

GILBREATH, B., and CICCHETTI, D. *Psychopathology in maltreating mothers.* Unpublished manuscript, 1990.

HARTUP, W. Peer relations. In P. Mussen, ed., *Handbook of Child Psychology.* Wiley, 1983.

HERTZBERGER, S. Social cognition and the transmission of abuse. In D. Finkelhor, R. Gelles, G. Hotaling, and M. Straus, eds., *The Darkside of Families: Current Family Violence Research.* Sage, 1983.

HESSE, P., and CICCHETTI, D. Toward an Integrative Theory of Emotional Development. *New Directions for Child Development* (1982) 16:3–48.

HOFFMAN-PLOTKIN, D., and TWENTYMAN, C. T. A multimodal assessment of behavioral and cognitive deficits in abused and neglected preschoolers. *Child Development* (1984) 55:794–802.

HOWES, C., and ESPINOSA, M. P. The consequences of child abuse for the formation of relationships with peers. *Child Abuse and Neglect* (1985) 9:397–404.

HUNTER, R. S., and KILSTROM, N. Breaking the cycle in abusive families. *American Journal of Psychiatry* (1979) 136:1320–22.

JACOBSON, R., and STRAKER, G. Peer group interaction of physically abused children. *Child Abuse and Neglect* (1982) 6:321–27.

KAUFMAN, J., and CICCHETTI, D. The effects of maltreatment on school-aged children's socioemotional development: Assessments in a day camp setting. *Developmental Psychology* (1989) 25:516–24.

KAUFMAN, J., and ZIGLER, E. The intergenerational transmission of child abuse. In D. Cicchetti and V. Carlson, eds., *Child Maltreatment: Theory and Research on the Causes and Consequences of Child Abuse and Neglect* Cambridge University Press, 1989.

KAZDIN, A. E., MOSER, J., COLBUS, D., and BELL, R. Depressive symptoms among physically abused and psychiatrically disturbed children. *Journal of Abnormal Psychology* (1985):298–307.

KEMPE, C. A practical approach to the protection of the abused child and rehabilitation of the abusing parent. *Pediatrics* (1973) 51:804–12.

KOTELCHUCK, M. Child abuse and neglect: Prediction and misclassification. In R. H. Starr, eds., *Child Abuse Prediction.* Ballinger, 1982.

LAHEY, B., CONGER, R., ATKESON, B., and TREIBER, F. Parenting behavior and emotional status of physically abusive mothers. *Journal of Consulting and Clinical Psychology* (1984) 52:1062–71.

LYNCH, M., and CICCHETTI, D. Patterns of relatedness in maltreated and nonmaltreated children: Connections among multiple representational models. *Development and Psychopathology* (1991) 3:207–26.

LYONS-RUTH, K., REPACHOLI, B., McLEOD, S., and SILVA, E. Disorganized attachment behavior in infancy: Short-term stability, maternal and infant correlates. *Development and Psychopathology* (1991):3.

MAIN, M., and GEORGE, C. Response of abused and disadvantaged toddlers to distress in agemates: A study in the day care setting. *Developmental Psychology* (1985) 21:407–12.

MAIN, M., and GOLDWYN, R. Predicting rejecting of her infant from mother's representation of her own experience: Implications for the abused–abusing intergenerational cycle. *Child Abuse and Neglect* (1984) 8:203–17.

MAIN, M., and SOLOMON, J. Discovery of a disorganized/disoriented attachment pattern. In T. B. Brazelton and M. W. Yogman, eds., *Affective Development in Infancy.* Ablex, 1986.

MAIN, M., and SOLOMON, J. Procedures for identifying infants as disorganized/disoriented during the Ainsworth Strange Situation. In M. Greenberg, E. Cicchetti, and M. Cummings, eds., *Attachment*

During the Preschool Years. University of Chicago Press, 1990.

MUELLER, N., and SILVERMAN, N. Peer relations in maltreated children. In. D. Cicchetti and V. Carlson, eds., *Child Maltreatment: Theory and Research on the Causes and Consequences of Child Abuse and Neglect.* Cambridge University Press, 1989.

ORNITZ, E. M., and PYNOOS, R. S. Startle modulation in children with Posttraumatic Stress Disorder. *American Journal of Psychiatry* (1989) 146: 866–70.

PARKE, R. D., and COLLMER, C. W. Child abuse: An interdisciplinary analysis. In E. M. Hetherington, ed., *Review of Child Development Research*, Vol. 5. University of Chicago Press, 1975.

PELTON, L. Child abuse and neglect: The myth of classlessness. *American Journal of Orthopsychiatry* (1978) 48:608–17.

PELTON, L. *Children Who Don't Want to Live.* Jossey-Bass, 1988.

PYNOOS, R. S., FREDERICK, C., NADER, K., ARROYO, W., STEINBERG, A., ETH, S., NUNEZ, F., and FAIRBANKS, L. Life-threat and posttraumatic stress in school-age children. *Archives of General Psychiatry* (1987) 44:1057–63.

REISS, D. *The Family's Construction of Reality.* Harvard University Press, 1981.

RIEDER, C., and CICCHETTI, D. Organizational perspective on cognitive control functioning and cognitive-affective balance in maltreated children. *Developmental Psychology* (1989) 25:382–93.

RODINO, P. W., Jr. Current legislation on victim assistance. *American Psychologist* (1985) 40:104–06.

ROSENBAUM, A., and O'LEARY, D. Marital violence: Characteristics of abusive couples. *Journal of Consulting and Clinical Psychology* (1981) 49:63–71.

ROSENBERG, M. S. New directions for research on the psychological maltreatment of children. *American Psychologist* (1987) 42:166–71.

RUTTER, M., and GILLER, H. *Juvenile Delinquency: Trends and Perspectives.* Penguin, 1983.

SAMEROFF, A., and CHANDLER, M. Reproductive risk and the continuum of caretaking causalty. In F. Horowitz, ed., *Review of Child Development Research*, Vol. 4. Chicago: University of Chicago Press, 1975.

SANTOSTEFANO, S. *A Bio-Developmental Approach to Clinical Child Psychology.* Wiley, 1978.

SANTOSTEFANO, S. *Cognitive Control Therapy with Children and Adolescents.* Pergamon Press, 1985.

SCHNEIDER-ROSEN, K., BRAUNWALD, K., CARLSON, V., and CICCHETTI, D. Current perspectives in attachment theory: Illustration from the study of maltreated infants. In I. Bretherton and E. Waters, eds., *Growing Points in Attachment Theory and Research.* Monographs of the Society for Research in Child Development 50, (Serial No. 209) 1985, pp. 194–210.

SCHNEIDER-ROSEN, K., and CICCHETTI, D. The relationship between affect and cognition in maltreated infants: Quality of attachment and the development of visual self-recognition. *Child Development* (1984) 55:648–58.

SCHNEIDER-ROSEN, K., and CICCHETTI, D. Early self-knowledge and emotional development: Visual self-recognition and affective reactions to mirror self-images in maltreated and non-maltreated toddlers. *Developmental Psychology* (1991) 27: 471–78.

SCHWARZ, E. D., and KOWALSKI, J. M. Malignant memories: PTSD in children and adults after a school shooting. *Journal of the American Academy of Child and Adolescent Psychiatry* (1991) 30: 936–44.

SIGEL, I. E. Reflections on the belief-behavior connection: Lessons learned from a research program on parental belief systems and teaching strategies. In R. D. Ashmore and D. M. Brodzinsky, eds., *Thinking About the Family: Views of Parents and Children.* Lawrence Erlbaum Associates, 1986.

SROUFE, L. A. Relationships, self, and individual adaptation. In A. Sameroff and R. Emde, eds., *Relationship Disturbances in Early Childhood.* Basic Books, 1989.

SROUFE, L. A., and FLEESON, J. Attachment and the construction of relationships. In W. Hartup and Z. Rubin, eds., *Relationships and Development.* Lawrence Erlbaum Associates, 1986.

SROUFE, L. A., and FLEESON, J. The coherence of family relationships. In R. A. Hinde, and J. Stevenson-Hinde eds., *Relationships within Families.* Clarendon Press, 1988.

STERNBERG, K. J., LAMB, M. E., GREENBAUM, C., CICCHETTI, D., DAWUD, S., CORTES, R. M., KRISPIN, O., and LOREY, F. *Developmental Psychology* (in press).

STRAUS, M. Cultural and organizational influences on violence between family members. In R. Prince and D. Barried, eds., *Configurations: Biological and Cultural Factors in Sexuality and Family Life.* Heath, 1974.

STRAUS, M., and GELLES, R. Societal change and family violence from 1975 to 1985 as revealed by two national surveys. *Journal of Marriage and the Family* (1986) 48:465–79.

STRAUS, M. A., GELLES, R. J., and STEINMETZ, S. K. *Behind Closed Doors: Violence in the American Family.* Anchor Press, 1980.

TERR, L. C. Psychic trauma in children: Observations following the Chowchilla school-bus kidnapping. *American Journal of Psychiatry* (1981) 138: 14–19.

TERR, L. C. Childhood traumas: An outline and overview. *American Journal of Psychiatry* (1991) 148: 10–20.

TOTH, S. L., MANLY, J. T., and CICCHETTI, D. Child maltreatment and vulnerability to depression. *Development and Psychopathology* (1992) 4:97–112.

TRICKETT, P. K., ABER, J. L., CARLSON, V., and CICCHETTI, D. The relationship of socioeconomic status to the etiology and developmental sequelae of physical child abuse. *Developmental Psychology* (1991) 27:148–58.

TRICKETT, P. K., and KUCZYNSKI, L. Children's misbehaviors and parental discipline in abusive and nonabusive families. *Developmental Psychology* (1986) 22:115–23.

TRICKETT, P. K., and SUSSMAN, E. J. Parental perceptions of childrearing practices in physically abusive and nonabusive families. *Developmental Psychology* (1988) 24:270–76.

TROY, M., and SROUFE, L. A. Victimization among preschoolers: The role of attachment relationship history. *Journal of the American Academy of Child Psychiatry* (1987) 26:166–72.

VAN DER KOLK, B. A. The separation cry and the trauma response: Developmental issues in the psychobiology of attachment and separation. In B. A. van der Kolk, ed., *Psychological Trauma*. American Psychiatric Press, 1987.

VONDRA, J. I. Sociological and ecological risk factors. In R. T. Ammerman and M. Hersen, eds., *Children at Risk: An Evaluation of Factors Contributing to Child Abuse and Neglect*. Plenum, 1990.

VONDRA, J., BARNETT, D., and CICCHETTI, D. Perceived and actual competence among maltreated and comparison school children. *Development and Psychopathology* (1989) 1:237–55.

VONDRA, J., BARNETT, D., and CICCHETTI, D. Self-concept, motivation, and competence among preschoolers from maltreating and comparison families. *Child Abuse and Neglect* (1990) 14:525–40.

WOLFE, D. A. Child abusive parents: An empirical review and analysis. *Psychological Bulletin* (1985) 97:462–82.

ZIGLER, E. Controlling child abuse: An effort doomed to failure? In W. A. Collins, ed., *Newsletter of the Division on Developmental Psychology, American Psychological Association*, February 1976, pp. 17–30.

ZIGLER, E. Controlling child abuse: Do we have the knowledge or the will? In G. Gerbner, K. Ross, and E. Zigler, eds., *Child Abuse: An Agenda for Action*. Oxford University Press, 1980.

The Horror! The Horror! Reflections on Our Culture of Violence and Its Implications for Early Development and Morality

Robert N. Emde

THIS commentary draws on two dimensions of chronic community violence, with thoughts that have been mobilized by the foregoing contributions. One concerns the importance of culture and the other concerns the importance of thinking about early development. Culture permeates all of our actions, and we are in a culture of violence. In other papers in this issue, Richters and Martinez point out that the United States is the most violent country in the industrialized world, and Ciccheti and Lynch state that violence "is becoming a defining characteristic of American society." We are fascinated by violence and in an implicit way we love violence–a fact that we need to acknowledge. Our fascination with violence in American culture is permeating and deep, and, as horrible as it is, I believe we need to face it in order to try to counter it.

I was reminded of this permeating dimension of our culture as I arrived at the hotel for the conference from which these papers emerged. On the table in my room was a magazine. It was a guide to cable TV and on its cover was a man who was pictured with a rather strained, smiling expression who looked at you with a clinched fist. The caption said, "Murder! A Battery of Killer Films! Assault TV!," trying to excite the reader. A number of films were then listed and at the bottom it added: "Plus . . . the small screens 20 biggest murders ever!" More than a decade ago, while studying abroad in London, I had similar thoughts about our American cultural fascination and our implicit acceptance of violence. One could walk rather freely in London at that time without the same kind of fear of guns and other violence that are typical of many U.S. cities. During that time, the news came that our president had been the victim of an assassination attempt. His remarks at the time were reported and positively connoted as reflecting his equanimity and good grace. The remarks did reflect these qualities, but I found them nonetheless shuddering, as I did the reaction of many in the United States. The wounded president's statement to the press, "I forgot to duck," also reflected a gamesmenlike quality along with what some interpreted as expectations of violence and murder.

One more illustration. On the day of my putting together this commentary, the *Sunday Denver Post* began the series "Kids and Guns" (see Roberts and Lipsher 1992). The text reports interviews from many who are carrying guns. Among the quotes, a 16-year-old girl says, "Everybody knows somebody who has a gun and car-

Robert N. Emde, MD, is supported in part by the National Institute of Mental Health project grant MH22803, Research Scientist Award 5 K02 MH36808, and the John D. and Catherine T. MacArthur Foundation Network in Early Childhood Transitions.

ries it. . . . its just the way it is now." Many talk about the meaning of the power of having a gun. A 17-year-old, speaking of the .38 semiautomatic he carried 2 years earlier stated, "It was like my Mom . . . it protected me." Another quote: "Whenever I go out with some of my friends, someone has a gun with them, a .22 or a .25. . . . there's always occasions to use them. We do drive-bys mostly or shoot them at the air or at a dog or any car that passes by." A girl, age 15, stated, "There's really nothing to learn about a gun . . . all you need to do is make sure it's with you and it's loaded. The only time you have it on 'safety' is when you're in your own house or a relative's house." Guns are readily available in Denver as in most other American cities—inexpensively bought or, as with young children, often obtained from parents. (Note a similar theme about gun availability shown on national television recently when CBS's "60 Minutes" portrayed the use of guns by young children.)

Unless we become aware of our fascination and acceptance of guns and violence, we will not have the opportunity to investigate alternatives, let alone mobilize the will for change. I will return to this theme in my conclusion.

A second dimension of my commentary concerns early development and morality. Our research group has constructed a theoretical model of early development that incorporates recent infancy research. We envision a set of inborn basic motives that are activated within the context of consistent caregiving that in turn lead to exploration, learning, and internalized shared meaning. These basic motives portray the infant as fundamentally active, self-regulating, and social, and as monitoring experience according to what is pleasurable and unpleasurable. Moreover, from the start, the infant explores the environment, seeking what is new in order to make it familiar (Emde 1988; Emde, Biringen, Clyman, and Oppenheim 1991). Our theory also describes how, in the course of everyday routines of consistent caregiving, basic motives become organized into more complex motives. Among these are: (1) the consolidation of an "affective core of self" that gives the infant a patterned sense of consistency through developmental change (Emde 1983), (2) derived relationship motives that give the infant a sense of wanting to repeat what is familiar in particular relationship experiences (Sander 1985), and (3) early moral motives.

Early moral motives are a consequence of internalizations that take place within the context of caregiving. Such internalizations have to do with the "dos" of experience as well as "don'ts." A brief consideration of what we have come to appreciate about infants raised in relatively low-stress environments forms a background for thinking about early development in the midst of chronic community violence.

The infant typically learns a great variety of "rules" as a shared aspect of the caregiving experience, before there is conflict and quite naturally as a positive aspect of such experience. These learned or internalized rules have a dual origin, including both: (1) an inborn propensity for initiating, maintaining, and terminating social interactions; and (2) expectable caregiver relationship experiences. Intricate sets of rules that govern "reciprocity" in face-to-face turn-taking interactions and other forms of communication operate well before language develops (for example, note documentations in Brazelton and Als 1979; Bruner 1982; Kaye 1982; Stern 1977; Trevarthen 1979; Tronick 1980). These developments are rudiments for a basic form of morality. All systems of morality are centered around reciprocity with some version of The Golden Rule: "Do unto others as you would have them do unto you." Moreover, a tendency for turn-taking in communication and for social cooperation may also be connected developmentally to another positive feature of early morality, namely, empathy. Toward the end of the child's second year, the infant typically comes to feel distress at another's expressed discomfort and may show a propensity to want to help or comfort the other (Radke-Yarrow, Zahn-

Waxler, and Chapman 1983; Zahn-Waxler and Radke-Yarrow 1982).

Toward the end of the second year, another feature of what we consider to be "basic morality" becomes differentiated. The tendency for "getting it right" about the world expresses itself in a new affective way. When faced with a familiar object that is flawed or dirty, the child sometimes shows anxiety when internal standards or expectations are violated. The child may evidence distress along with an urge to correct what is perceived as a discrepancy (Dunn 1988; Kagan 1981). Kagan has highlighted this developmental milestone to the onset of reflective self-awareness and has emphasized that all systems of morality require internalized standards – along with a sense of uneasiness when prototypic standards are violated.

Thus our theory proposes that by the end of the second year a child has elements of a basic positive morality, by virtue of internalizing the dos of everyday interactions with caregivers. An internalized sense of reciprocity, a sense of everyday rules (for example, about what to do, when to do it, and what belongs where), empathy, and some internalized standards are part of this development. Typically, affect plays a major role as pleasure in "getting it right," which is confirmed by the caregiver's expression of pride and as lingering experiences of shame and disappointment in the course of interactions also begin to have a role.

The child's internalizing of don'ts also occurs through repeated interactions with caregivers. Observations of caregiver–infant interactions during the child's second year highlight processes of social referencing and negotiation in mediating self-regulation. Social referencing occurs when the child encounters situations of uncertainty and the child seeks out emotional information from a significant other in order to resolve the uncertainty and to regulate behavior. Thus, when a stranger approaches or a strange toy is presented, the child will look to the caregiver and if the latter smiles or expresses interest, the re-sult will be encouragement to explore and touch; if the caregiver expresses fear or anger, the child will tend to avoid the new situation. We find a similar searching for emotional signals during situations when prohibitions are given by caregivers. Repeated looking occurs following vocalized prohibitions, and the child seeks a resolution of uncertainty or a confirmation for a decision about acting. Indeed, we have found that negotiation in the context of repeated prohibitions makes use of social referencing in this way and leads to internalized procedures for moral (and self) regulation. Typically, negotiation occurs when parents offer initially unclear emotional messages (depending on the context of what is prohibited), along with mild prohibitions; these messages are then "tested" by the infant. Sequences of such experiences are then internalized and made use of in subsequent encounters. We tend to say that shared meaning is negotiated in the course of back-and-forth exchanges with significant others; the young child thereby comes to internalize strategies of action with particular others in varying contexts. Thus, more than we had imagined, early development is revealed to be creative; it not only involves processes of construction on the part of the child and coconstruction on the part of the child-with-caregiver, but it also involves the child's internalizing remarkably dynamic experiences and procedures of negotiation.

Longitudinal observations indicate that by the end of the second year, children typically show evidence of having internalized rules for don'ts; they evidence restraint in the midst of prohibitions so long as the caregiver is physically present and available for social referencing. Internalization of don'ts without the parent being present in the midst of temptation, however, requires further development. Such development may also depend upon the acquisition of moral scripts that have narrative and emotional coherence: an acquisition that occurs during the child's third year and beyond (Buchsbaum and Emde 1990).

Although direct research has not been done with respect to such processes in the context of chronic community violence, the foregoing contributions in this issue suggest some stark realities and their consequences. In this issue, the picture drawn by the work of Richters and Martinez, as well as that of Osofsky, Wewers, Hann, and Fick, and that of Bell and Jenkins, give indication of the devastating effects of the violent scene on caregiving – whether in Washington, DC, New Orleans, or Detroit. Such effects necessarily lead to caregiver restriction of activity in young children in order to ensure safety and survival. Garmezy commented that mothers who keep their children safe in our besieged urban ghettos are the unacknowledged moral heroes of our time (Garmezy 1991). Still, one wonders about the restricted breadth of values, goals, attitudes, and aspirations that must necessarily occur from the decreased developmental opportunities under such circumstances. As Friedlander has pointed out in his contribution to this issue, chronic violence undermines the child's potential basic trust and sense of reliable support for learning, as well as the child's potential sense of security because of unresolvable fear. In addition to fear, one can add the stresses of loss and grief that are likely to disrupt everyday interactions of caregivers; all of these stresses are likely to lead to a relative deficit of opportunities for internalizing experiences of reciprocity, to a restriction of opportunities for internalizing a variety of "rules and expectations," and to a restriction of opportunities for experiencing empathy, repairs, and other kinds of positive shared meaning.

But one also wonders about other kinds of risks for development along these lines. In addition to deficit, one wonders about deviant developmental pathways. What are the different kinds of expectations and goals along with later kinds of internalized scenarios that will develop in young children in such an atmosphere of chronic fear, loss, and restriction? In this issue, the contribution of Lorion and Saltzman comments on the general desensitization to threat and even addictive risk-taking behavior that can develop later under these circumstances.

Research has not yet been done that can give us direct knowledge about such influences from chronic violence. But research has been done on influences from family violence and child maltreatment. In this issue, the contributions of Cicchetti and Lynch and of Putnam and Trickett document findings with respect to distortions of emotional regulation that can occur in the child in such circumstances. Children and adults can suffer a variety of disturbances in affiliation and reciprocity in different social relationships, including those involving peers, spouses, and parenting. Putnam and Trickett comment on potential psychophysiological consequences related to elevated cortisol responses to chronic stress and its possible influences on neuronal loss. This also puts this commentator in mind of recent advances in our knowledge of early brain development, wherein we have learned there is normally on overproduction of cells and synapses with functional connections that undergo a "pruning" during early development. Although it is a matter of some scientific debate, early experiences and functional use may have a role in determining which synaptic connections and pathways "survive" in the brain (Edelman 1987).

In concluding, I would like to mention what we have recently come to refer to as a "Jeffersonian Principle" of early moral development (Emde and Clyman In preparation). The rudiments of early moral development, according to our view, take place procedurally, before the acquisition of language and before internalized knowledge can be represented in declarative fashion. Early internalized rules are not represented consciously, even though they come to govern behavior in coherent ways. Thus, rules about the way the world is and should be, as well as rules about reciprocity and tendencies to repair internalized standards that are discrepant from one's expectations, are based on procedural knowledge and are nonconscious. In the course of later development, these rudiments become part of a more complex process of "getting it right about the world." But they persist. And here we come to our Jeffersonian principle. There is a sense, as Thomas Jefferson put it, of internalized "truths" that we hold to be "self-evident." The evocation of this phrase, from the founding days of our Republic, also brings with it Jefferson's predications: "among these are life, liberty, and the pursuit of happiness." What opportunities do young children suffering from chronic community violence in the U.S. today have for such predication? What truths do they hold as self-evident? Jefferson's framework for our thinking brings us back to the opening theme of my commentary. This concerns our coming to grips with our culture of violence today and its consequences for moral development. My title is taken from Coppola's movie, "Apocalypse Now," and from Joseph Conrad: "The Horror! The Horror!" But acknowledging the horror in ourselves and in our circumstances, means that we have both incentive and opportunity to tap another feature of our American culture and democracy – mainly that of optimism and a willful activity to overcome adversity. Friedlander, in his contribution, points out that we have made significant progress with respect to national social problems such as in stigmatizing smoking and advancing women's rights. The problem we are addressing in this issue of *Psychiatry* is every bit as urgent.

REFERENCES

BRAZELTON, T. B., and ALS, H. Four early stages in the development of mother-infant interaction. *Psychoanalytic Study of the Child* (1979) 34:349-69.

BRUNER, J. S. *Child's Talk: Learning to Use Language*. Norton, 1982.

BUCHSBAUM, H. K., and EMDE, R. N. Play narratives in thirty-six-month-old children: Early moral development and family relationships. *Psychoanalytic Study of the Child* (1990) 40:129-55.

DUNN, J. *The Beginnings of Social Understanding*. Harvard University Press, 1988.

EDELMAN, G. M. *Neural Darwinism: The Theory of Neuronal Group Selection*. Basic Books, 1987.

EMDE, R. N. The prerepresentational self and its affective core. *Psychoanalytic Study of the Child* (1983) 38:165-92.

EMDE, R. N. Development terminable and interminable: I. Innate and motivational factors from infancy. *International Journal of Psycho-Analysis* (1988) 69:23-42.

EMDE, R. N., BIRINGEN, Z., CLYMAN, R. B., and OPPENHEIM, D. The moral self of infancy: Affective core and procedural knowledge. *Developmental Review* (1991) 11:251-70.

GARMEZY, N. Community Violence and Children's Development: Conference Report and Photo Essay by David E. Scharff. *Washington School of Psychiatry, Update and Catalog of Events* (Winter 1991) 2(4):20.

KAGAN, J. *The Second Year: The Emergence of Self-Awareness*. Harvard University Press, 1981.

KAYE, K. *The Mental and Social Life of Babies: How Parents Create Persons*. University of Chicago Press, 1982.

RADKE-YARROW, M., ZAHN-WAXLER, C., and CHAPMAN, M. Children's prosocial dispositions and behavior. In P. H. Mussen, ed., *Handbook of Child Psychology*, 4th ed., E. M. Hetherington, ed., Vol. 4. Wiley, 1983.

ROBERTS, J. A., and LIPSHER, A. (April 12, 1992). Kids and Guns. *The Sunday Denver Post*.

SANDER, L. Toward a logic of organization in psychobiological development. In K. Klar and L. Siever, eds., *Biologic Response Styles: Clinical Implications*. Monograph Series of the American Psychiatric Press, 1985.

STERN, D. N. *The First Relationship: Mother and Infant*. Harvard University Press, 1977.

TREVARTHEN, C. Communication and cooperation in early infancy: a description of primary intersubjectivity. In M. Bullowa, ed., *Before Speech: The Beginning of Interpersonal Communication* (pp. 321-47). Cambridge, England: Cambridge University Press, 1979.

TRONICK, E. The primacy of social skills in infancy. In D. B. Sawin, R. C. Hawkins, L. O. Walker, and J. H. Penticuff, eds., *Exceptional Infant*, Vol. 4 (pp. 144-58). Brunner/Mazel, 1980.

ZAHN-WAXLER, C., and RADKE-YARROW, M. The development of altruism: Alternative research strategies. In N. Eisenberg, ed., *The Development of Prosocial Behavior*. Academic Press, 1982.

Impact of Violence on Children and Adolescents: Report from a Community-Based Child Psychiatry Clinic

Marilyn Benoit

THE Children's National Medical Center is located in the inner-city area of Washington, DC. As is nationally now well publicized, the drug-related violence in Washington has earned the area the dubious title of "murder capital of the world." Our outpatient child and adolescent psychiatry clinic at Children's Hospital provides walk-in services during daytime hours, Monday through Friday. Access to services is available at other times through the emergency room.

In my brief report I attempt to describe a cross-sectional sample of the violence-related cases that have been presenting to our walk-in clinic. This clinical presentation further supports what other papers in this issue report: that there is significant psychiatric morbidity associated with the public health menace we call violence. This crisis was summarized by a cartoon that was featured in the *Washington Post*'s "Drawing Board" (Marlette for *New York Newsday*): Two Black boys are shown in an urban setting, sitting on steps in the midst of gunfire. One asks the other, "What would you like to be when you grow up?' and the heartbreaking response is "Alive!" The cartoon captures the plight of many of our urban, minority, children. It indeed depicts an environment that most of us would consider a war zone. In Washington, DC, alone, the 1986 homicide rate was six times the national average (Shisana and Kofie 1990). In more understandable terms, this meant fewer than one homicide per day. In 1989 the rate was 1 homicide per day and in 1990 it

was greater than 1 per day. The 1991 homicide total was 496. The message of the *Washington Post* cartoon is all too poignant against such a statistical backdrop. From the six cases that follow, some common themes emerge—themes that dramatize how our inner-city children and youth are being psychologically victimized by the violence in our society.

CASE 1

This case is a 9.5-year-old African-American male with a history of father having been shot to death 5 months previously. He presented with the following symptoms:

- Sadness
- He fights when kids tease him about his father.
- Behavior problems in school and oppositional behavior at home.
- Wish to be "dead like father."
- He fears that someone could break into the house and hurt him.

Marilyn Benoit, MD, is Acting Chairperson, Department of Psychiatry, Children's National Medical Center; and Associate Professor, Department of Psychiatry and Behavioral Sciences and Pediatrics, The George Washington University, Washington, DC.

• Wants to be a policeman "to lock people up when they do something bad."

CASE 2

A 19-year-old Black female presented with a sleep disturbance. She has been withdrawn and fearful since the shooting death of her cousin, who was gunned down at his job. This woman also demonstrated:

• Difficulty separating from mother.
• Paranoid thinking.

CASE 3

This is a 5-year, 9-month-old African-American male refusing to go outside. He lives in a drug-infested and crime-ridden neighborhood. He has experienced the loss of two closely involved males, who were shot to death in his block. The fire engines and ambulance came to the neighborhood on both occasions. The child now shakes and clings to his grandmother when he hears a siren. The grandmother brought him to the walk-in clinic because she is concerned that the shootings in the neighborhood have affected him. Other pertinent information about this youngster include:

• Father is a drug addict and ex-convict who lives on the street.
• Mother's whereabouts are unknown.
• Teacher reports that he is petrified of the violence in the neighborhood.
• He talks a lot about guns and shooting.
• Likes to instigate fights and inflict pain.
• Appears sad and scared.
• Wants to become a policeman to save people.

CASE 4

This is a 8.5-year-old African-American male with neurovegetative symptoms and somatic complaints. Additional details include:

• Presence of suicidal ideation, but not intent.
• Onset 8 days after violent death of father, who was shot 7 times in the chest in drug-related murder.
• Child read newspaper report.
• He wants to seek revenge.
• He witnessed mother receiving a severe beating from second husband. She had to be hospitalized.
• Worried about house being broken into.
• Has been making weapons to protect himself.

CASE 5

This 16-year-old African-American male presented with deteriorating school performance. Further details include:

• Onset followed event when he and some friends were held up at gun point by four men who took one friend's jacket and threatened to kill him.
• He ran to the police but friends threatened to beat him up for running away.
• He is irritable, gets angry easily, and is scared to go anywhere alone.

CASE 6

This is an 18-year-old self-referred male who presented to walk-in with the following history:

• Previous day, policemen entered his home with guns pointed at the occupants, including himself.
• House was searched and all occupants were frisked.
• One person was allegedly beaten by police and taken to jail.
• That night, patient had difficulty sleeping because of nightmares and flashbacks.
• He described feeling sad, anxious, and fearful, and had no interest in food.

The literature on posttraumatic stress disorder emphasizes (Eth and Pynoos 1985, Terr 1979) the importance of early intervention and the need for mastery of the trauma. In the treatment of the patients presented here, the therapist has an extremely difficult challenge. In cases of physical or sexual abuse, the victim can be removed from the abusive environment. In the case of trauma following a natural disaster, the statistical probability of the same occurrence in the immediate future is generally quite low. However, these particular patients do not have the luxury of choice as regards relocating their households to nonviolent and costlier neighborhoods. They are faced with a very real sense of importance and a high probability of reexposure to violence in their neighborhoods. It seems that we must devote our efforts to primary prevention since our therapeutic intervention can be at best moderately palliative, not curative.

REFERENCES

ETH, S., and PYNOOS, R., eds. *Posttraumatic Stress Disorder in Children*. American Psychiatric Press, 1985.

SHISANA, O., and KOFIE, V. *Trend Analysis of Homicides in the District of Columbia, 1980–1989*. Research and Statistics Division, Office of Policy and Planning, Government of District of Columbia, 1990.

TERR, L. Children of Chowchilla. *Psychoanalytic Study of the Child* (1979) 34:547–623.

Children in Poverty: Resilience Despite Risk

Norman Garmezy

TWO objectives provided the focus for the Conference on Community Violence and Children's Development that was jointly sponsored by the National Institute of Mental Health and the John D. and Catherine T. MacArthur Foundation. One was to examine the evidence for deficit behaviors that characterized children reared in poverty; the second was to identify the characteristics of children who sustained their competencies despite being reared in comparable environments. These dual objectives took this form: "What can we conclude from studies of children, their families, and environments about characteristics that *predispose* children to maladjustment following exposure to violence, and about characteristics that *protect* children from such adjustment problems following, or in the midst of, violence exposure?"

Thus stated, the formulation placed the goals of the conference in the heartland of ongoing research on *risk* and *protective* factors that guide the behaviors of children in highly stressed environments – a central concern of those who have been associated with the emergent field of developmental psychopathology (e.g., Achenbach 1982; Cicchetti 1989; Lewis and Miller 1990; Masten, Best, and Garmezy 1990; Robins and Rutter 1990; Rolf et al. 1990; Sameroff and Emde 1989; Sroufe and Rutter 1984; Stevenson 1985).

Implicated in that search is a focus on those elements in person, family, community, and culture that may conduce to the development of adaptive or maladaptive behaviors. The ultimate test of such variations lies in the quality of functioning that can be observed in children exposed to life's stressors and trauma-inducing environments. "Risk" is the language of epidemiology with its emphasis on *actualized* risk that takes form in the manifestation of a disease process or disordered behavior. In comparison, research on the correlates of adaptive functioning under such stress experiences is of more recent origin (Garmezy 1985; Masten 1990; Rutter 1979, 1985, 1987). The suggestive evidence of the power of protective factors has begun to challenge investigators, but it remains a younger and less mature sibling to the older and more adequately studied effects stemming from actualized risk factors.

CUMULATED RISK

There are numerous examples of the effects generated by cumulative risk factors in psychiatric research. In studies conducted by Rutter and his colleagues both on the Isle of Wight and in an impoverished borough of London, Rutter (1979)

Norman Garmezy, PhD, is Professor Emeritus of Psychology, University of Minnesota.

I express my gratitude to my research colleagues at the University of Minnesota, Drs. Ann Masten and Auke Tellegen. Our work has been facilitated by the NIMH, the William T. Grant Foundation, the John D. and Catherine T. MacArthur Foundation, and by the Graduate School of the University of Minnesota.

identified six family-linked variables that when cumulated were significantly associated with an increased likelihood of psychiatric disorder in offspring: (1) severe marital discord, (2) low SES, (3) overcrowding or large family size, (4) paternal criminality, (5) maternal psychiatric disorder, and (6) foster home placement of the children in the family.

The findings demonstrate the powerful negative consequences attendant on the cumulation of these chronic adversities (Garmezy and Masten in press). Thus, the presence of a single stressor (or of no stressor at all) produced a 1% increment in psychiatric disorder in children. Two stressors in the family complex provided a 5% rise in the disorder rate; three stressors, a 6% increment; and four or more stressors accounted for a 21% increment in the rate of child psychiatric disorders. Thus the cumulative presence of stressors accounted for a 33% psychiatric rate, with multiple stressors accounting for the largest proportion of the disorders.

Similar findings have been evident in research conducted by Kolvin and his colleagues (1988a, 1988b, 1988c) in the longitudinal New Castle Family Study of risk factors and their influence on the development of later criminality. Their cumulative indicators paralleled those employed by Rutter: (1) marital instability, (2) parental illness, (3) poor domestic and physical care of the children and home, (4) dependency on state or community for subsistence, (5) overcrowded housing, and (6) poor mothering ability. Follow-up studies of the criminal records of the offspring revealed a marked relationship between summated adversities and rates of offending.

A third examination of the effects of cumulative exposure to risk elements was conducted by Sameroff and his colleagues (1982, 1984, 1989, 1990) in their studies of children born to schizophrenic mothers. Here the stressors numbered 10: (1) maternal mental illness; (2) high maternal anxiety; (3) mother's rigidity in attitudes, beliefs, and values regarding her child's development; (4) few positive maternal interactions with her child; (5) unskilled occupational status of the head of household; (6) minimal maternal education; (7) disadvantaged minority status; (8) reduced family support; (9) stressful life events in the family; and (10) large family size. Once again cumulation of these chronic adversities had a pronounced negative effect on the child's cognitive and social/emotional development. Sameroff has suggested that the presence of each adverse factor, in effect, cost the child 4 IQ points. It is evident that chronic familial adversities exercise a detrimental effect on many children so exposed (Garmezy and Masten In press).

The authors note that a parallel cofactor to these findings resides in the socioeconomic status of the nation. They had linked their children's performance, between ages 4 and 13, to changes that took place in the economic status of families. Describing a Congressional Report, Sameroff et al. (1989) point to the period between 1973 and 1987 (the time period in which the study was conducted) in which the average household income of the poorest fifth of Americans fell 12%, while the income of the wealthiest fifth in the nation increased 24%. If there is a sociopolitical aspect to the study of risk it may be found in these coinciding sets of data. But single explanatory factors do not suffice. Since Sameroff et al.'s study was focused on the offspring of schizophrenic mothers, it is likely that both biogenetic factors *and* social conditions may have jointly operated to heighten the risk status of children at biological disadvantage living in impoverished circumstances.

Chronic poverty provides a longitudinal account of cumulative stressors that begin with poor maternal health and inadequate nutrition for the impoverished pregnant mother. What follows often extends to inadequate obstetrical supervision, high rates of mortality and morbidity in the infant, and for some, malnutrition and illness that is often enhanced by a lack of adequate medical care. Later in the lives of many poor children there follows school failure, and in time an occupational history marked by low-level jobs, inadequate salaries, and often chronic unemployment. The transgenerational nature of these cumulative stressors (Birch and Gussow 1970) stretched over years disadvantages children and adults in poverty. It makes difficult the breaking of the chain sequence of stressors that confine the hopes and aspirations of the poor. That many escape is a tribute to the resilience of many people of poverty.

These findings reflect the downside of the linkage power of sociocultural and biological elements to affect potentially disadvantaged lives. But there is a positive side to the coin as well. For the data within the previously cited studies confirm that there are children who, despite their exposure to multiple risk factors, do not show the dire consequences that have been reported. Obviously, as risk factors pile up, the probability of a positive outcome is appreciably reduced. There is, however, a knowledge gap in our research focus, for only in recent years have investigators begun to explore the lives of similarly disadvantaged children for whom positive outcomes have been reported.

RESILIENCE AS A CONSTRUCT

For these children it is necessary to search for the presence of "protective" factors that presumably compensate for those "risk" elements that inhere in the lives and in the environments of many underprivileged children. Some have identified this task as the study of "resilient" or "stress-resistant" children. Others have chosen to use the more compelling identifier of "invulnerable" children (Anthony and Cohler 1987). I believe this latter designation is best avoided since it promises far more than most children can produce under the repetitive onslaught of cumulative stressors.

A comparison of definitions of these two words, "resilient" and "invulnerable," makes evident the distinction. "Resilience" as defined in the Oxford English Dictionary provides a metaphoric representation for this aspect of human behavior: "the tendency to rebound or recoil," "to return to a prior state," "to spring back," "the power of recovery." There is a functioning flexibility associated with "resilience" not accorded to "invulnerable" with its definition properties: "incapable of being wounded or injured," "not liable to be physically hurt or damaged," "not effectively assailable." Clearly the term "resilience" captures what is meant when one speaks of a person who regains functioning following upon adversity. Thus "to spring back" does not suggest that one is incapable of being wounded or injured. Metaphorically, it is descriptively appropriate to consider that under adversity, an individual can bend, lose some of his or her power and capability, yet subsequently recover and return to the prior level of adaptation. The prior position presumably is one that reflects certain competencies and it is to this state that the resilient person returns as stress is reduced or compromised. The central element in the study of resilience lies in the power of recovery and in the ability to return once again to those patterns of adaptation and competence that characterized the individual prior to the prestress period.

In a recent review of research on resilience in childhood, Luthar and Zigler (1991) have examined a number of studies that have reported on the issue of the continuity over time of disadvantaged children's resilient behaviors. In citing the findings of Farber and Egeland (1987), the authors report that levels of competent functioning in abused and neglected children tested five times between the ages of 12 and 42 months indicated that there was a subset of children who appeared competent at each testing occasion. However, their numbers tended to decline over time, leading the investigators to suggest that a continuation of abuse in the home may have been responsible for a decline in functioning. This study may provide another example of the negative power of cumulated stressful experiences.

Such results should not be surprising. Indeed these reports actually strengthen the case for "resilience" in opposition to "invulnerability." If all adults are presumed to have a "breaking point," then why not children? And why not subsequent recovery for many if, and when, stressful conditions have eased?

Two other studies raise a related issue. Farber and Egeland (1987) have suggested that within their sample of young children there are a number who show competent behavior and good coping strategies but who are not "emotionally healthy." Behavioral competence, Luthar and Zigler (1991) suggest, is not necessarily paralleled by superior adjustment in all spheres of functioning, including freedom from anxiety, distress, and other internalizing states.

Similarly, Werner and Smith (Werner 1989; Werner and Smith 1982, 1992), in their justifiably famed study of the children of Kuaia, have indicated that at age 30, when 62 of the original sample of 72 resilient children were again evaluated, good coping with adult responsibilities was evident, but this was not accompanied in all cases by happiness or life satisfaction. Werner (1989) reported that some of the resilient males have had difficulty in establishing committed intimate relationships in adulthood. Further, health problems seemingly related to stress have also been observed.

These findings provide new questions and new avenues for research. What factors are involved in the seeming diminution over time of resilience in some hitherto adaptive children and adults? Prolonged and cumulated stress would appear to be a prime candidate for examination. Another factor worthy of consideration would be the absence of a support structure and its availability over time. Other candidates for affecting change may be critical modifications in the child's environment such as the physical dissolution of the family.

Clearly, what is needed are intensive studies of these shifts in individual adaptations and a search for their correlates. These might take the form of short-term longitudinal studies focused around critical transition periods in development. Clinical and experimental studies of children who show such adaptational changes would warrant a search for modifications in the child's status, family and friendship losses, school failures, etc.

A cautionary note is in order. Signs of emotional distress do not necessarily suggest a breakdown in resilient behavior. Manifestations of competent functioning must still be evaluated. In our Project Competence research program (now under the direction of Dr. Ann Masten), we continue to monitor competence indicators over time, looking to individualized aspects of our case history analyses to classify competent functioning in the domains of family, school, and peers using diverse assessment strategies, ranging from intensive interviews to specific test situations. These studies, which emphasize a search for competence indicators, have been conducted over three testing points spread over a 12- to 13-year period.

Our definition of a competence item is one that measures successes and achievements in meeting the major adaptational expectations or requirements for people of the age of our subject in society. For older adolescents and young adults these would include: academic and job performance, obedience to law, expectations for appropriate social conduct with adults (e.g., parents, teachers, employers), relating well to peers, having a close relationship with a friend, preliminary signs of developing romantic relationships (e.g., dating), etc. (Coatsworth 1991).

In the absence of such a vigorous research and clinical effort, caution is needed before assuming the adaptive status of an individual. I would hold to the position that emotional distress per se would not nullify the copresence of resilient behavior in child and adult. While examples of this position are scarce in the literature of childhood, it is manifestly evident in adult performance. War with exposure to combat provides an exemplar of an almost universal fear and emotional distress accompanied in most instances by the retention of functional behavior.

Research during World War II demonstrated a similar adaptability of children during the London Blitz. In the presence of their parents and given supportive parental behavior, the children of London rode out the firestorm. However, these observations do not negate the necessity of a careful consideration of those additional attributes of adaptability that comprise the nature of resilience in children.

It may seem paradoxical that manifest competence and emotional disturbance can coexist in some children. Such patterns in children's reactions to stress represents a challenge to researchers and clinicians alike, and suggests a direction in research that hitherto has been neglected.

FOSTER CARE AND LATER ADAPTATION

The paradox has been evident in a volume appropriately titled: *No One Ever Asked Us* (Festinger 1983). This volume reports a follow-up study of the adult outcomes of 277 persons placed in foster care early in their childhood in New York City, because of neglect, parental mental illness, abandonment and desertion, parental inability to cope, or physical illness or death of the parent.

These children, placed early in childhood, were kept in that status until they were released to the community, with relatively little preparation, when they had reached their maturity. The reasons for the placement of these children emphasized their at-risk status. These included neglect (24%), mental illness of the primary caregiver (20%), parental inability to cope (12%), abandonment and desertion by the parent (12%), physical illness (8%), and death of the parent figure (6%). In only 2.5% of the cases was the child's behavior the cause of the placement.

Further, placement instability and discontinuities marked the "travels" of many of these children who had been assigned to foster homes or institutional settings. In the former cases some 68% had three or more different placements, which often occurred among the 3- to 4-year-olds.

Descriptively, the children were designated as Black (51.7%), White (27.7%), Hispanic (19.1%), and Oriental (1.5%). Festinger indicates that the biological parents tended to be at the "lower rungs of the socio-economic ladder" as indexed by their limited education, poor occupational histories, and scanty financial resources. Divorce and separation was the lot of many of these parents.

Clearly, here was a high-risk group, a factor repeatedly cited when Festinger asked others to predict the post-foster home adaptation of this cohort. Most cited negative outcomes, but these predictions proved false.

Festinger (1983) compared the statuses of the 277 young adult men she subsequently located with a subset of family-reared controls of the same age and sex drawn from a national survey conducted by the Institute of Social Research at the University of Michigan. The groups of foster-reared children and the comparison group of young adults were rated in terms of their friendships, achievements, and employment rates. Although the foster group showed lower scholastic achievements, their employment rates were similar for White respondents within the two groups and somewhat lower for the Black adults. In terms of health and symptom status the groups were similar; so too were their personal evaluations of their feelings, their future hopes, and their current sense of happiness.

Clearly the dreaded expectations about the adult adaptations of these foster-reared children were not fulfilled. Nor was there an excessive dependence in this group on welfare or on receiving public support. Festinger notes that the foster-placed groups were generous contributors to the study; they exhibited a willingness and an openness to discuss their lives in the hope that it would help others.

Festinger concludes her volume with a query: "Why," she asks, "[is there] such a singular emphasis on vulnerability? [Why] . . . so little confidence in young people's capacities to come to grips with the reality that no one's world is perfect?

Why so little faith in the strength and resilience of children?" (p. 253).

CHILD ABUSE AND LATER ADAPTATIONS

Child abuse is another area that warrants attention because of the powerful belief that continuity into adulthood characterizes the transition of the abused child to the adult abuser. Unfortunately, there are comparatively few longitudinal studies of the long-term outcomes in child abuse cases. A study conducted in Israel by Zimrin (1986) gives pause in asserting an invariant continuity from abused to abuser. The number of cases studied is small but the period of follow-up covers 14 years of the group of 28 abused children into late adolescence and early adulthood. Zimrin notes that a "survivor" group did not succumb to a sense of hopelessness as their inevitable fate. They believed they could achieve and set out to do it.

They did not carry with them the excess baggage of being stupid or worthless. They did not exhibit manifest psychiatric disturbances; they were neither suicidal nor self-destructive. They had good and in some cases outstanding intellectual talents. In terms of hopes and fantasy, they maintained a positive outlook on life, turning away from despair, passivity, defeatism, or yielding behavior. Indeed, at times they were provocative and demanded attention. Their presenting picture was not an entirely happy one but there was evident a certain toughness and resilience in these early-abused children. An important factor in their survival was their cognitive attainments. There remains, notes Zimrin, a "gamut of problems" evidenced by the survivors including a lack of ability to express emotion, and an isolation and a difficulty in interpersonal relationships. However, these adaptive adolescents are not dysfunctional in terms of aggression, hopelessness, or the abuse of others. An anticipated longer-term follow-up will provide a portrait of their adaptation in adulthood.

PROTECTIVE FACTORS AMIDST ADVERSITY

The evidence is sturdy that many children and adults do triumph over life's adversities. What then are the possible "protective factors" that enable individuals to overcome life's stressors? There are hints in the literature that suggest the variables that may be operative and adaptive in meeting stressful life situations.

In an early search of a scanty literature (Garmezy 1985), three factors seemed to be recurrent: (1) the modification of stressors by potential *temperament factors*, including activity level, reflectiveness, cognitive skills, and a positive responsiveness to others; (2) *families*, including those in poverty, marked by warmth, cohesion, and the presence of some caring adult such as a grandparent who takes responsibility in the absence of responsive parents or in the presence of strong marital discord; (3) the presence of some source of *external support* as seen in the presence of a strong maternal substitute. This can be a teacher, a neighbor, parents of peers, or even an institutional structure such as a caring agency, a church, etc.

When this triad was first formulated by a focus on a very small and diverse literature, it was suggested as a tentative and potentially unreliable statement. It has, however, been strengthened by the reports of Werner (1989), who characterized a subset of resilient adults whom she studied in a follow-up into adulthood of her Children of Kuaia. Werner wrote:

Three types of protective factors emerge from our analyses of the developmental course of high-risk children from infancy to adulthood: 1) dispositional attributes of the individual, such as activity level and sociability, at least average intelligence, competence in communication skills (language and reading), and an internal locus of control; 2) affectional ties within the family that provide emotional support in times of stress, whether from a parent, sibling, spouse, or mate; and 3) external support systems whether in school, at work, or church, that reward the individual's competencies and determination, and provide a belief system by which to live. (p. 80)

The critical role of family has been noted by other investigators (e.g., Clark 1983; Comer 1980; Williams and Kornblum 1985). The significance of schools and teachers is a recurrent theme in the literature of "school climate" and its importance in the development of cognitive and social skills in poor children (Brookover et al. 1978; Comer 1980; Mortimore et al. 1988; Neisser 1986; Rutter et al. 1979). The critical importance of the maintenance of institutions and role models within the ghetto has been set forth in a highly significant volume by Wilson (1987).

All these represent the gradual emergence of factors that influence resilience in children in disadvantaged settings and under disadvantaging circumstances. But this is only a beginning, for the important research that must follow is the discovery and elaboration of the mechanisms and processes that underlie resilient behaviors in children under stress (Garmezy 1991; Rutter 1987). Once we have identified the biological, psychological, and sociocultural mechanisms that activate resilient behavior and the developmental processes that are integral to the operation of these mechanisms, we will then be in a better position to generate scientifically sturdy programs of intervention that may enable us to develop methods for enhancing resilient behavior in children disadvantaged by status and stress.

The Science and Politics of Resilience

Two tasks now challenge us. One is scientific, the other political. First, to the scientific agenda. Confirmatory studies are needed to invigorate the reality that in America's city ghettos and rural farm communities, wherever poverty is manifestly evident, a substantial core of America's poor children, likely a majority, possess a potential for achievement that must be nurtured and expanded. We must learn more about the patterning of functions in these children and the factors

housed in person, family, and community that are precursors to their survivorship. The person factor will implicate biology, genetic, and social-developmental elements in which sociocultural factors, family belief systems and values, and parent–child relationships will be vital components.

To this must be added the role of community and the broader environment of the child. Part of the community will be the opportunity structure provided for the child beginning with schools and the climate for learning afforded the child. The literature of school climate and its relationship to the acquisition of needed skills is a powerful one. *Fifteen Thousand Hours* (Rutter et al. 1979) details the attributes of good versus poor schools located in an inner borough of London marked by poverty. This research emphasizes such elements as a positive school climate, including concerned teachers and principals, parents who are active participants in the school's goals, and a setting where safety is transcendant and pupils share some responsibility for the quality and enterprise of the school. In such settings, Rutter et al. reported that children profit, their examination scores are positive, and their rates of employment and their maintenance of employment 1 year following graduation differ significantly from less adequate schools in the same deprived neighborhoods.

Parallel studies in the United States are supportive. The efforts of James Comer (1980) have made evident the positive effects gained when a favorable school climate is advanced by the collaboration of parents, teachers, and administrators despite a school's location in disadvantaged neighborhoods. In this context the school can be a major protective factor; in negative contexts, schools add to the cumulation of stressors associated with poverty.

There are other protective factors worthy of study. In terms of biological individuality there is the critical role played by temperament—an elusive construct given the heterotypic continuity associated with various temperaments as manifested at later points in the life cycle. The intellective component, embraced by IQ, is another critical factor, as is the presence of a cohesive, warmly supportive family, one that can be generated by a single parent and not solely in dual-parent households.

Since we are in the midst of a powerful biological revolution, I feel the need to assert that protective factors are not biolog-free zones of scientific inquiry. Traits, temperaments, intelligence, all share biological underpinnings. Family care, too, undoubtedly links to a history of gene and environment, as does long-term intergenerational stability. But these biological propensities are not the sole province of middle- and upper-class life. Children of the ghetto and their parents share in those biological and social-psychological attributes that enhance survivorship.

Support systems, about which much has been written in recent years (Antonucci 1990; Cohen and Syme 1985; Kahn and Antonucci 1980; Kessler et al. 1985; Riley and Eckenrode 1986), also may have a biosocial interactive component. The strivings of a child, the manifestation of motivation, the setting of goals, etc., may well predispose an adult to extend support to the child, to foster involvement and helpfulness. This tentative view, however, bears a requirement of proof and verification.

The focus on resilience amidst disadvantage also carries a political component, for the problem of poverty is a vital aspect of the political agenda of the nation. If family cohesion, children's adaptation, and the utility of support systems are components of family survivorship in economic adversity, then these must be joined to a nation's manifest concern for the poor. The nation's recent test of "benign neglect" has brought only failure and an increase in the intensity that surrounds the issues of rural and urban poverty. The Conference on Violence and Children's Development where the papers in this issue were first presented is an example of the effort to undo the consequences of such neglect. In taking the liberty to politicize this conference I invoked the Japanese

tradition of the red kimono. It is my understanding that in Japan, once you pass age 70, you are free to put on the kimono and thus speak freely about pressing events.

In the content area of this conference, the political issue and the scientific agenda cannot be discrete entities; they link together in enhancing not only scientific knowledge but also that which lies within the domain of government's concern for its underprivileged citizens. We need research support for continuing studies of children at risk for psychiatric disorder, of children introduced early in their lives to violence on the streets, and to the attractiveness of crime. For the psychiatrically disordered, we must develop ways of alleviating the heavy, cumulative burden of risk factors, that four-plus exposure and its consequences suggested by Rutter, Kolvin, Sameroff, and others. At the same time we need financial support for interventions to shore up the manifest talents of children and families of the ghetto who do not present the problem of cumulative risk, but whose danger is accentuated by the threatening ecologies in which they reside.

This conference, with its emphasis on both deficiency and adaptability of children in poverty, is very important for comprehending the current national crisis. What must be borne in mind is that there are heroes out there who need assistance – mothers determined to save their children; mothers who stand on the stoops of apartment buildings in our inner cities peering down the dangerous streets to watch their children coming home from school.

I carry with me a story told to our MacArthur Foundation Network on Successful Adolescence in High-Risk Settings by two distinguished ethnographers, Drs. Terry Williams and William Kornblum. It is a story of competence and concern in a Harlem neighborhood in New York City. In the foyer of a walkup apartment building there was a large frame on the wall within the entrance way. The photographs of children who lived in the apartment building were pasted on the frame with a written request that if anyone saw any of these children endangered on the street to bring them back to the apartment house. My thoughts focus on those who conceived the idea, put up the sign, and joined in providing photographs of their children. Can there be a better example of adult competence and concern for the safety of children? Is this effort not a dramatic reflection of what we mean when we seek to describe "protective" factors on behalf of the well-being of children under stress? And most important of all, should not our nation's concern extend to ensuring the safety of these children, the well-being of their families, and thus, the well-being of our country?

There is a duty that this nation has to all of its children, namely to ensure the maximization of their talents. Thomas Jefferson provided a historical perspective and a path to that maximization. In setting forth a plea and a plan for universal public education, Jefferson in 1783 in his *Notes on Virginia* wrote:

By that part of our plan which prescribes the selection of the youths of genius among the classes of the poor, we hope to avail the state of those talents which nature has sown so liberally among the poor as of the rich, but which perish without use if not sought for and cultivated.

That act of cultivation reflects the basic ethos of the nation. In that act lies the beginning of solutions to many of the social problems that now beset our society.

REFERENCES

ACHENBACH, T. *Developmental Psychopathology*, 2nd ed. Wiley, 1982.

ANTHONY, E. J., and COHLER, B. J., eds., *The Invulnerable Child*. Guilford Press, 1987.

ANTONUCCI, T. C. Social supports and social relationships. In R. H. Binstock and L. K. George, eds., *Handbook of Aging and the Social Sciences*, 3rd ed. (pp. 205–27). Academic Press, 1990.

BIRCH, H. G., and GUSSOW, J. D. *Disadvantaged Children: Health, Nutrition and School Failure*. Harcourt, Brace and World, 1970.

BROOKOVER, W. B., SCHWEITZER, J. H., SCHNEIDER, J. M., BEADY, C. H., FLOOD, P. K., and WISENBAKER, J. K. Elementary school climate and school achievement. *American Educational Research Journal* (1978) 15:301–18.

CLARK, R. M. *Family Life and School Achievement: Why Poor Black Children Succeed or Fail*. University of Chicago Press, 1983.

CICCHETTI, D., ed. *The Emergence of a Discipline: Rochester Symposium on Developmental Psychopathology*. Lawrence Erlbaum, 1989.

COATSWORTH, J. D. *Continuities and discontinuities in competence from middle childhood to late adolescence*. Doctoral dissertation, University of Minnesota, 1991.

COHEN, S., and SYME, S. L., eds., *Social Support and Health*. Academic Press, 1985.

COMER, J. P. *School Power*. Free Press, 1980.

FARBER, A. E., and EGELAND, B. Invulnerability among abused and neglected children. In E. J. Anthony and B. J. Cohler, eds., *The Invulnerable Child* (pp. 253–88). Guilford Press, 1987.

FESTINGER, T. *No One Ever Asked Us*. Columbia University Press, 1983.

GARMEZY, N. Stress-resistant children: The search for protective factors. In J. E. Stevenson, ed., *Recent Research in Developmental Psychopathology*. Journal of Child Psychology and Psychiatry Book Supplement. (1985) 4:213–33.

GARMEZY, N. Resiliency and vulnerability to adverse developmental outcomes associated with poverty. *American Behavioral Scientist* (1991) 34: 416–30.

GARMEZY, N., and MASTEN, A. M. Chronic adversities. In M. Rutter, L. Hersov, and E. Taylor, eds., *Child and Adolescent Psychiatry*, 3rd ed. Blackwell Scientific Publications, in press.

KAHN, R. I., and ANTONUCCI, T. C. Convoys over the life course: Attachment, roles and social support. In P. B. Baltes and O. Brim, eds., *Life-Span Development and Behavior* (1980) 3:254–83.

KESSLER, R. C., PRICE, R. H., and WORTMAN, C. B. Social factors in psychopathology: Stress, social support, and coping processes. *Annual Review of Psychology* (1985) 36:531–72.

KOLVIN, I., MILLER, F. J. W., FLEETING, M., and KOLVIN, P. A. Social and parenting factors affecting criminal offence rates: Findings from the Newcastle Thousand Family Study, 1947–1980. *British Journal of Psychiatry*, (1988a) 152:80–90.

KOLVIN, I., MILLER, F. J. W., FLEETING, M., and KOLVIN, P. A. Risk and protective factors for offending with particular reference to deprivation. In M. Rutter, ed., *Studies of Psychosocial Risk: The Power of Longitudinal Data* (pp. 77–95). Cambridge University Press, 1988b.

KOLVIN, I., MILLER, J. F. W., SCOTT, D. McI., GATZNIS, S. R. M., and FLEETING, M. *Adversity and*

Destiny: Explorations in the Transmission of Deprivation—Newcastle "1000" Families Study. Gower, 1988c.

LEWIS, M., and MILLER, S. M., eds., *Handbook of Developmental Psychopathology.* Plenum, 1990.

LUTHAR, S. S., and ZIGLER, E. Vulnerability and competence: A review of research on resilience in childhood. *American Journal of Orthopsychiatry* (1991) 61:6–22.

MASTEN, A. S. Resilience in development: Implications of the study of successful adaptation for developmental psychopathology. In D. Cicchetti, *The Emergence of a Discipline* (pp. 261–94). Lawrence Erlbaum, 1990.

MASTEN, A. S., BEST, K. M., and GARMEZY, N. Resilience and development: Contributions from the study of children who overcome adversity. *Development and Psychopathology* (1990) 2:425–44.

MORTIMORE, P., SAMMONS, P., STOLL, L. LEWIS, D., and ECOB, R. *School Matters: The Junior Years.* Open Books Publishing, 1988.

NEISSER, U. *The School Achievement of Minority Children: New Perspectives.* Lawrence Erlbaum Associates, 1986.

RILEY, D., and ECKENRODE, J. Social ties: Subgroup differences in costs and benefits. *Journal of Personality and Social Psychology* (1986) 51:770–78.

ROBINS, L., and RUTTER, M., eds., *Straight and Devious Pathways from Childhood to Adulthood.* Cambridge University Press, 1990.

ROLF, J., MASTEN, A. S., CICCHETTI, D., NUECHTERLEIN, K. H., and WEINTRAUB, S., eds., *Risk and Protective Factors in the Development of Psychopathology.* Cambridge University Press, 1990.

RUTTER, M. Protective factors in children's responses to stress and disadvantage. In M. W. Kent and J. E. Rolf, *Primary Prevention of Psychopathology,* Vol. 3: *Social Competence in Children* (pp. 49–74). University Press of New England, 1979.

RUTTER, M. Resilience in the face of adversity: Protective factors and resistance to psychiatric disorder. *British Journal of Psychiatry* (1985) 147:598–611.

RUTTER, M. Psychosocial resilience and protective mechanisms. *American Journal of Orthopsychiatry* (1987) 57:316–31.

RUTTER, M., MAUGHAM, N., MORTIMORE, P., and OUSTON, J. *Fifteen Thousand Hours.* Harvard University Press, 1979.

SAMEROFF, A. J., BAROCAS, R., and SEIFER, R. The early development of children born to mentally ill women. In N. F. Watt, E. J. Anthony, L. C. Wynne, and J. E. Rolf, eds., *Children at Risk for Schizophrenic: A Longitudinal Perspective* (pp. 482–514). Cambridge University Press, 1984.

SAMEROFF, A. J., and EMDE, R. D., eds., *Relationship Disturbances in Early Childhood: A Developmental Approach.* Basic Books, 1989.

SAMEROFF, A. J., and SEIFER, R. Early contributors to developmental risk. In J. Rolf, A. S. Masten, D. Cicchetti, K. H. Neuchterlein, and S. Weintraub, eds., *Risk and Protective Factors in the Development of Psychopathology* (pp. 52–66). Cambridge University Press, 1990.

SAMEROFF, A. J., SEIFER, R., BALDWIN, C., and BALDWIN, A. *Continuity of risk from early childhood to adolescence.* Presented at the biennial meetings of the Society for Research in Child Development, Kansas City, 1989.

SAMEROFF, A. J., SEIFER, R., and ZAX, M. Early development of children at risk for emotional disorder. *Monographs of the Society for Research in Child Development* (1982) 47(7).

SROUFE, L. A., and RUTTER, M. The domain of developmental psychopathology. *Child Development* (1984) 83:173–89.

STEVENSON, J. E., ed., *Recent Research in Developmental Psychopathology.* Pergamon Press, 1985.

WERNER, E. E. High-risk children in young adulthood: A longitudinal study from birth to 32 years. *American Journal of Orthopsychiatry* (1989) 59:72–81.

WERNER, E. E., and SMITH, R. S. *Vulnerable but Invincible: A Study of Resilient Children.* McGraw-Hill, 1982.

WERNER, E. E., and SMITH, R. S. *Overcoming the Odds.* Cornell University Press, 1992.

WILLIAMS, T., and KORNBLUM W. *Growing up Poor.* Lexington/D. C. Heath, 1985.

WILSON, W. *The Truly Disadvantaged.* University of Chicago Press, 1987.

ZIMRIN, H. A profile of survival. *Child Abuse and Neglect.* (1986) 10:339–49.